THE COMPASSIONATE PRACTITIONER

by the same author

Transformation through Journal Writing
The Art of Self-Reflection for the Helping Professions
Jane Wood
ISBN 978 1 84905 347 1

Inspiring Creative Supervision
Caroline Schuck and Jane Wood
ISBN 978 1 84905 079 1
eISBN 978 0 85700 271 6

of related interest

Relating to Clients
The Therapeutic Relationship for Complementary Therapists
Su Fox
ISBN 978 1 84310 615 9
eISBN 978 1 84642 718 3

How to Incorporate Wellness Coaching into Your Therapeutic Practice
A Handbook for Therapists and Counsellors
Laurel Alexander
ISBN 978 1 84819 063 4
eISBN 978 0 85701 034 6

Archetypal Imagery and the Spiritual Self
Techniques for Coaches and Therapists
Annabelle Nelson
ISBN 978 1 84819 220 1
eISBN 978 0 85701 169 5

Shamanism and Spirituality in Therapeutic Practice
An Introduction
Christa Mackinnon
ISBN 978 1 84819 081 8
eISBN 978 0 85701 068 1

THE COMPASSIONATE PRACTITIONER

HOW TO CREATE A SUCCESSFUL AND REWARDING PRACTICE

JANE WOOD

ILLUSTRATIONS BY JANE WOOD

SINGING
DRAGON

LONDON AND PHILADELPHIA

First published in 2014
by Singing Dragon
an imprint of Jessica Kingsley Publishers
73 Collier Street
London N1 9BE, UK
and
400 Market Street, Suite 400
Philadelphia, PA 19106, USA

www.singingdragon.com

Library of Congress Cataloging in Publication Data
A CIP catalog record for this book is available from the Library of Congress

British Library Cataloguing in Publication Data
A CIP catalogue record for this book is available from the British Library

ISBN 978 1 84819 2 225
eISBN 978 0 85701 170 1

Printed and bound in Great Britain

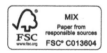

CONTENTS

ACKNOWLEDGEMENTS

My thanks and gratitude to everyone who has encouraged me to write this book, and especially to those who have given me their suggestions, feedback and personal experiences. Particular thanks go to Mike and Linda for their proofreading and to Dave for his thought-provoking comments. It has been a privilege to teach and supervise the many practitioners who have contributed to my understanding of the practitioner–patient relationship.

My loving appreciation to my family for their encouragement, technical support and proofreading.

INTRODUCTION

In the dark before dawn
joyful after winter storms
a blackbird sings

(Wood, unpublished)

The Compassionate Practitioner is a book written for independent, self-employed practitioners. It centres on the importance of a trusting relationship between practitioner and patient. This is a temporary relationship created solely for the work of helping the patient using a specific therapy or modality. The practitioner–patient relationship does not replace the therapy or become therapy in itself – but rather creates a strong foundation upon which the therapy can be practised. Without a trusting relationship there can be a lack of commitment on both sides leading to non-returning patients and a frustrated practitioner.

A really effective consultation is more than a series of questions and answers. A lot goes on non-verbally as the practitioner strives to understand the patient, and the patient in turn assesses whether they can trust the practitioner. What the patient is looking for is respect, compassion and understanding.

In *The Compassionate Practitioner* every stage of the consultation is examined carefully, considering both the practitioner's and patient's needs. There is a lot you can do to prepare in advance of the patient arriving. When they have arrived you can begin with making the patient feel comfortable and safe by creating a working agreement and clarifying the boundaries. Once these needs are satisfied, you can start the case-taking using the wide variety of skills and techniques explained here. Finally you can wind down the session, discuss your findings with the patient, and negotiate the way forwards.

It sounds simple enough, doesn't it? Yet in my research into different alternative therapies over the years, my experience has shown me first-hand how the relationship can be mishandled. There are few good role models around. Sadly, in orthodox medicine, the short consultation times and group practices make logistical and financial sense, but make creating a relationship with each patient increasingly difficult.

When a nourishing practitioner–patient relationship is set up, everyone benefits. The patient feels respected and understood and is more likely to return for further appointments, which exponentially increases their chance of healing. The practitioner gains in experience and confidence, and the whole practice begins to flourish and expand.

Two parallel themes run throughout the book, those of mindfulness and compassion. Mindfulness means bringing your awareness to the present moment and reducing other thoughts, such as the previous patient or the lunch to come. If you practise mindfulness it has several consequences. You will feel calmer and less stressed in your work, because you will have learnt to slow down the busy chatter of your thoughts. When you are mindful during the case taking you will focus more on the case and listen wholeheartedly. This allows you to see the case more clearly and understand what needs to be cured. The patient will appreciate both your calmness and your attentive awareness.

Compassion is about feeling the patient's pain or suffering and allowing this understanding to inform the treatment. It links the patient's story to the universal human experience, taking away all prejudice or blame. Compassion can also be given to yourself, as you tell yourself to let go of the stranglehold of perfection, and be content as the 'good enough' practitioner. Self-compassion is not the same as self-pity which has an element of helplessness. Instead self-compassion is coupled with learning, which keeps you on the road moving forward.

A third theme runs throughout *The Compassionate Practitioner*, and that is of self-reflection. This is the art of looking objectively at your work and examining it in order to learn from yourself. To keep self-reflection from becoming a record of self-criticism and self-defeat, you should look at both your strengths and your weaknesses. Then you can appreciate all of your successes, however small they are, as well as learn from your mistakes and failures. Self-reflection balances self-compassion and ensures growth in the practitioner, contributing to your continuing practitioner development (CPD). Self-reflection can be done with a supervisor or by yourself using a journal dedicated to the purpose. At the end of each chapter in this book there is a journal example.

The Compassionate Practitioner was a book that demanded to be written, coming from my 20 years as a practitioner, teacher and supervisor as well as my research and my experience in the patient role. I wanted to write this book for all those alternative practitioners who have invested so much time and money into studying their therapy, yet have found building up their practice to be slow and unrewarding. I wanted to show how success is built up layer by layer, starting with the practitioner's attitude towards themselves, their patients and their practice.

Above all this is a practical book, full of advice and suggestions about how to create a flourishing practice without exhausting yourself or giving less to your patients. There is a chapter on self-care, suggesting many ways to relax in your time off and avoid burnout. Becoming a wholehearted practitioner is a work in progress, forever expanding, developing and learning from your experience.

This book was written for alternative practitioners of all disciplines, but it will be of interest to anyone who is in the helping professions or studying to become so. It will be of value to complementary and alternative practitioners such as homeopaths, acupuncturists, shiatsu practitioners, Chinese medicine practitioners, naturopaths, nutritional therapists, Reiki practitioners, body-workers and herbalists. It could also benefit art, music and drama therapists.

I have used the words 'practitioner' and 'therapist' to mean the person who provides the healing modality, and the word 'therapy' to describe their discipline. All of the cases are made up but they are inevitably influenced by my 20 years' experience as a practitioner and as a supervisor. The book can be either read through from start to finish or dipped into at random.

My hope is that by introducing more rigour into the way that they approach the practitioner–patient relationship, alternative practitioners can become more professional. This will make their patients feel safer and more respected and the practitioner will feel free to express their compassion. Everyone will gain, and the practice will flourish.

Chapter 1

THE POWER OF POSITIVE THINKING

When I first started practice in 1990, advertising meant renting space in the local newspaper or alternative health magazine, putting your business card in the newsagent's window or giving talks. Since then the expansion of technology has opened up ever-increasing methods of getting yourself known. I haven't written about the new technology – it would be out of date before the book is published – but I do suggest it takes more than advertising and networking to be successful. It is your positive attitude that will bring you patients, job satisfaction and success.

Many alternative practitioners have a negative attitude about success in their practice. They graduate with optimism, but soon enough their inner voice is telling them that it is difficult, they won't make enough money, they haven't got enough time, they can't find a good clinic room and so on. They begin to hope for the best but prepare for the worst; unfortunately these two cancel each other out.

One of the best ways to change your attitude is by working with the self-reflective journal. This is a handwritten or on-screen journal that is kept specifically for writing down and exploring work-related issues, with a view to understanding them and yourself in relation to them. Gradually you can open up some of your unconscious thoughts, attitudes, beliefs or prejudices, and decide whether you want to keep these for the future or make changes. When you understand yourself better, you can consciously choose to be more positive and actively seek success. There is an example of a self-reflective journal at the end of each chapter in this book. Chapter 13 is dedicated to keeping a journal.

FOCUSING ON YOUR SUCCESS

Quite early on in my career as teacher and supervisor, I recognized that many adult learners are extremely good at listing their weaknesses and failures but find it difficult to acknowledge or appreciate their success. It is as if success is only deemed noteworthy if it is A-grade or higher. For those who are studying to enter the caring professions, there are further pitfalls waiting. Students can easily find themselves measuring their success by the well-being of their patient or client rather than also looking inward and congratulating themselves on the good work they have done.

The human brain has a natural tendency to look at the negative aspects first. Martin Seligman (2011), writing in *Flourish, a New Understanding of Happiness and Well-Being – And How to Achieve Them*, explains:

> For sound evolutionary reasons, most of us are not nearly as good at dwelling on good events as we are at analyzing bad events. Those of our ancestors who spent a lot of time basking in the sunshine of good events, when they should have been preparing for disaster, did not survive the Ice Age. So to overcome our brains' natural catastrophic bent, we need to work on and practise this skill of thinking about what went well. (p.33)

In Britain, thinking or talking about personal success is often avoided as we have been taught that it is selfish, boastful, egocentric or just bad manners. Whilst I agree that continuously talking about your own success to others could be considered all of these, acknowledging a job well done to yourself or to a critical friend can be affirming and satisfying. A critical friend is someone like a close colleague, who understands your work and you can trust. An agreement is set up between you so you can challenge and support each other.

A student arranged to do some online supervision with me. She had low self-confidence and often believed she was not good enough as a practitioner. She had very high standards and expected a lot of herself. I suggested that when she was writing in her journal, she included the two reflective questions, *What did I do well?* and *What didn't I do so well?* I told her that it is important to congratulate yourself on any success you have, however small. If you celebrate what you have done well as a practitioner you will be more likely to repeat your good or effective behaviour, and over time you will consolidate good practice. If you only reflect on what you didn't do so well, you will lower your self-confidence.

The student began working this way, and in her self-reflections started to include phrases such as, 'I acknowledge my ability to...,' Or, 'I am consciously aware of accepting myself.' I was pleased with this beginning, but I felt that her comments were rather lukewarm and encouraged her to be more enthusiastic. In the following reflection, she experimented by telling herself that she was proud of her work with a difficult patient in clinic. She found it was such an unusual experience that she questioned why she should be uncomfortable with self-praise. The answer came easily: self-praise had elements of arrogance and ego, and as a child she had been taught that boasting was not nice. She didn't want to be seen as arrogant or boastful.

I explained to her that there is a difference between boasting in front of others, and congratulating yourself in a reflective journal or in the privacy of your thoughts, for a piece of work that has been done well. The former is done in order to gain rank or status above others. The latter is done privately as part of a balanced assessment of your experience.

A key moment for me was when I ran a two-day workshop with my Japanese students on the practitioner–patient relationship. As we approached the last segment of the weekend, I spontaneously decided to end the workshop with a self-appreciation session. I sat all of the participants in a circle, and asked them to pass around the microphone, so that one by one they could state what they had done well over the weekend and what they had not done so well. For the first five or six people, this appeared excruciating. They were willing enough to blame themselves, but far too polite to praise themselves in public. In some cases I had to enlist the help of those that had worked with them in order to find something praiseworthy. Gradually, as we went around the circle, the later students began to loosen up, dared to be honest and even raised sympathetic laughter as they admitted they hadn't expected to do so well.

After this I challenged all my students to write both *What went well* and *What didn't go so well* in their reflective journals. My decision was at first instinctive but gradually I built up a rationale, described here in my book, *Transformation through Journal Writing*:

I am a strong advocate of including both positives and negatives in a journal. The self-reflective journal will be a necessary recipient of problems, dilemmas, upsets and failures. It is through working on these issues that a writer can begin to understand themselves and initiate change. If these issues are not brought into the journal, the writer is being superficial and will not claim the reward of self-development. However, if the journal writer is continuously being self-critical it will lower their self-esteem… If strengths and weaknesses are both given page space in the journal, the writer feels a sense of balance. (Wood 2012, p.72)

Writing about your successes helps you identify your strengths, boosts your self-confidence, and encourages you to repeat successful behaviour. The self-reflective journal should be something that supports you as well as being a learning aid. It should contain enough positives so that you enjoy rereading it. Beyond the description of what went well, the same spirit of inquiry can be brought to a positive issue as a negative issue. If something went well, how do you feel about it? What was your attitude of mind leading up to the positive outcome? Would there be value in repeating this experience in other contexts? (Wood 2012, p.73)

Concentrating on your success does not mean being blind to your faults, nor does it mean waiting for a major breakthrough before you can celebrate. It means acknowledging fairly what you did well, however small it was. It is human nature to notice what mistakes you made and where you went wrong, and these will need working on so that you don't repeat them. Just remember it is also human nature that being told off makes you feel bad and being praised makes you feel good. So praise yourself for the little things, such as making the patient feel comfortable, ordering the supplies you forgot last time, cleaning your desk, doing your filing or getting an appreciative thank you after a treatment.

SUCCESS ATTRACTS MORE SUCCESS

According to the Law of Attraction, we can directly influence what comes into our lives through our thoughts, emotions and intentions. This has been written about since the beginning of the last century and proposes that whatever comes to us is a direct reflection of what energy we give out. Losier (2007) writing in *Law of Attraction: Getting More of What You Want and Less of What You Don't*, defines it as: 'I attract into my life whatever I give my attention, energy and focus to, whether positive or negative' (p.12). If this is the case, then it is definitely worth giving attention and energy to what is positive, in order to get more of the same. Every small success that is acknowledged and celebrated will attract more success.

An example of Law of Attraction working is the newly qualified practitioner who wants to build up a private practice. The tendency is often to think in terms of 'not enough patients' which leads to negativity, maybe even to self-blame. According to the Law of Attraction, the more they become anxious and think about not-enough (experience, knowledge, patients, money, publicity, etc.), the less they will get. The Law of Attraction will quite simply provide them with more of the not-enough state because that is what they are focusing on. This means it doesn't help to look at reality and bemoan that it has not changed. In order to attract what it is you really want, you need to turn your attention to thoughts and emotions about your vision of how it will be. This can be done either through visualization, or thinking/writing with pleasure about each small success as it happens.

It takes a conscious effort to change your thinking; it will not happen spontaneously and has to be worked on. Imagine each part of your body can contribute towards your thinking mind, instead of imagining the mind as a single organ placed somewhere in the brain. What if every part of your body has a voice and together they create an endless, semi-conscious chatter with input from first one part and then another, constantly changing direction? Sometimes it feels as if these background thoughts are in control of you, but they are not who you really are. You can step outside of them and quieten them using regular meditation, and they can be deliberately changed from negative to positive.

The first step is to change the thinking from 'not enough' to 'plenty of', and remind yourself of this as frequently as possible throughout the day. It would feel strange and untrue to jump directly from 'not enough' to 'plenty of' so it needs to be practised using some softening and soothing words, such as: 'Wouldn't it be nice to have plenty of (patients, money, time, etc.). It feels good to imagine plenty, I like the thought of plenty, I like the thought that it would be easy to get plenty. There are other areas of my life that are abundant and I would like abundance in my career as well' (see Figure 1.1). If there is time to do a dedicated visualization of the 'plenty of', choose a medium that resonates with you. Is it best to do this in your head, out loud, as a drawing or in writing? Some people are more comfortable with words and others more comfortable with images. Some people like to sing. Do you prefer to do it alone or with a witness?

More than just thinking in words about success, your emotions need to be included as well. Try smiling while you are congratulating yourself for what you've done well. The brain automatically links smiling with happiness, and it doesn't matter which comes first. Happiness produces smiles and smiles produce happiness. Remind yourself of all the things that have gone well, where you have had success and felt good. These don't have to be A-grade or gold-star occasions; just remember the feeling of riding your bicycle or driving your car for the first time, going on holiday and getting your first glimpse of the sea, or receiving your first pay cheque. Remember the grin on your face, the feeling of dancing excitement inside, the silly things that you did to celebrate and the laughter.

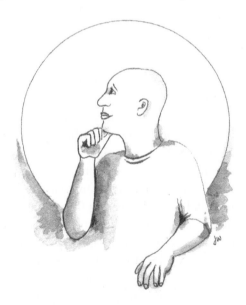

FIGURE 1.1: DAYDREAM YOUR FUTURE SUCCESS

POSITIVE VISUALIZATION

Positive visualization clarifies your intention of what you really want so you can concentrate your energies in that direction. It is best done when you are in a cheerful state of mind. If you try doing it while you're feeling negative, you can end up giving conflicting messages of hope and doubt. Visualization is a clear statement of wanting change, but if it's coupled with a negative state of mind you might cancel out any benefits.

If you're feeling positive while doing a visualization, then you can be very specific about what you want. However, being specific can put a lot of pressure into the mix. It highlights what you really do want, but at the same time it inevitably emphasizes what you haven't got, making the visualization seem like a futile exercise. Also, if all your criteria are set in stone, it prevents further creativity.

It is far better is to be general and look at the underlying feeling or sensation that will be experienced once the desired results have been achieved. A visualization that is general rather than specific usually connects more easily with the feelings and sensations rather than the facts. If you want to build up your practice, you should consider what it would feel like to have a flourishing practice. Perhaps you feel a smiling satisfaction that your skills are increasing with experience, or the thrill of excitement as your diary fills up. Maybe you have a feeling of empowerment as your confidence builds up or a feeling of peace and calmness.

A visualization that I sometimes do in workshops is to consider the doorway to your clinic. Sit comfortably cross-legged or with both feet on the floor and be quiet for a while. Focus on your breathing and try to reduce the number of thoughts whirling around in your mind. In your imagination, see your clinic doorway as a magic portal into a parallel world, where you are welcoming a queue of new patients coming to see you. There is a big smile on your face, your hands are beckoning them in and you are greeting them with loving kindness and respect. When you have completed the visualization, get a large piece of paper and some coloured pens and draw yourself standing in the doorway with your words of cheerful welcome around you. You might write phrases like, 'It's great to see you,' 'I'm looking forward to working with you,' 'Come inside, you're very welcome' or 'Thank you for recommending me to other patients.'

PRACTICAL VISUALIZATION

Not all visualizations need to be in the mind. For some people it is easier to write it out as a rambling monologue, an organized list or a growing mind map. Maybe the visualization only clarifies for you when your fingers touch the keyboard or your pen meets paper. Perhaps it is easier for you to draw or paint the feeling in colours. Words are not always necessary.

Sometimes doing something practical acts as a visualization, simply because it focuses your mind on your work. Checking over your equipment, washing the covers of your treatment couch, ordering new supplies or making some positive change to the appearance of your clinic room are all done with the underlying message that new patients will be coming.

I always found that when my practice was slow it would help to spend the time doing some spring cleaning or space clearing in and around my clinic room. This is both practical and an effective visualization. I didn't need to calculate what sort or how many new patients I wanted. That would have been too specific. I just needed to make space for several new people. I would sweep the path to my clinic room, symbolically inviting new patients to access me easily. I would wash the clinic door, and buy some flowering plants to put in the garden. I might tidy up my bookcase, throw away unnecessary papers from my desk or create more space in my filing cabinet for the new patients I was expecting.

KNOW YOUR OWN STRENGTHS

Martin Seligman (2011) writing about the positive psychology movement, emphasizes the need to replace negative thinking with positive. He describes working with depressed patients and realizing that even if he could take away all of their negative emotion, the patient would be left in an empty state, not a positive one. The patient has to learn the skills of being positive. He writes:

> If we want to flourish and if we want to have well-being, we must indeed minimize our misery; but in addition we must have positive emotion, meaning, accomplishment, and positive relationships. (p.53)

In the same way, if you have practised negative thinking since childhood, judging and blaming yourself for not being good enough, you will need to build up your total confidence. Even a simple task like routinely writing down six positive experiences that happened during the day, every evening, will slowly contribute to your overall sense of well-being. If you go to sleep feeling pleased with six things that went well, you are more likely to wake up feeling cheerful.

Seligman drew his conclusions from his research as a psychologist working with depressed people. Paul E. McGhee (1996) came to the same conclusion from the opposite direction. He researched humour for 20 years and writes in *Health, Healing and the Amuse System, Humour and Survival Training*:

> If you have a negative, pessimistic outlook on life, you can generally find things to justify it. After all life is full of injustice. And the more support you can find for your outlook, the more it feeds your pessimism. But if you make the effort, you can often find a positive, as well as a negative, aspect of the same bad situation. So you have a choice of focusing your attention on the negative or the positive. We've all heard about seeing the glass as 'half full' or 'half empty'. Which kind of person are you? (pp.129–130)

Seligman (2011) designed a questionnaire that helps people discover their strengths.[1] Seligman explains that when someone has truly identified their personal strengths, there is a sense of ownership and authenticity. They start to tailor every task according to their strengths, and knowing this, they feel excited, enthusiastic and invigorated. They want to use their strengths as much as possible, and get involved in personal projects that demand their strengths.

My own way of getting people to look at their strengths is less scientific. I suggest that you consider what else you bring to your job apart from the vocational skills, knowledge and experience that you have achieved. Instead, consider all the different unacknowledged skills that you have gained over the years through learning or experience. Below are some cue questions that might help you remember and acknowledge your strengths and qualities. You might come up with some negative things as well, but just for now please ignore them and simply turn your attention to the positive. This is your boasting list and should be written in large letters in your journal, or better still put up on the wall opposite where you sit. It should make you smile and feel proud of yourself:

- Think of all the exams you have taken over the years, including music exams, first aid courses and driving test.

---

1   The questionnarie can currently be found on www.authentichappiness.com (last accessed on 7 April 2014).

- Remember any specialist subject that you have learned, such as sailing, lacemaking, a new language or DIY, and decide what else it taught you.

- Think of all the skills that you have learned through sport or exercise.

- Cherry pick through your life experiences as a child and choose the positives that contribute to who you are now.

- Look at your life experiences as an adult and choose those that advanced your self-development.

- Consider the relationships you have had with family and extended family and think of what you have learnt from them.

- Remember any intensive time spent with different age groups, such as with a new baby or an elderly relative, and see what qualities this brought out in you.

- Review all of the jobs you have taken, and decide what you learned from them.

- Consider the skills that you developed when working in a team with classmates or colleagues.

As you reflect on the boasting list, acknowledge and praise yourself for what you do well. For example, 'I am very calm in a crisis,' 'I am really good at listening,' 'I have a passion for gardening and growing my own food' or 'I am very good at public speaking.' Notice the other skills and qualities that were brought out in you through your experiences. You might have learned the skills of teamwork or telesales, or acquired the values of tolerance or calmness. Even your childhood stubbornness might have developed into commitment and firmness of purpose.

Knowing your personal strengths goes far beyond celebrating each time you do something well, or visualizing more success. It gives you a personal toolkit that you can use with confidence whatever your ultimate goal. It gives you a self-identity that you can value, work with and feel positive about.

DEVELOP AN ATTITUDE OF SUCCESS

Success is more than following a formula and having a concrete result. It is not enough to advertise, network, link up and make new Internet friends. It depends upon your attitude and your energy. Feeling anxious about your weaknesses can send a subtle message to the people around you through your body language, facial expression, choice of words, strength of delivery and tone of voice. They will sense your doubt in yourself and they will doubt you in return. Choosing to look at the positive sides of your work and your personal strengths will contribute to your inner confidence and your outer success.

You have worked hard to get where you are, and now is the time to appreciate yourself. There are a lot of things you have done very well in the past, and if you didn't praise yourself then, do it now. Look in the mirror, look into your own eyes and tell yourself that you love yourself. Be kind and compassionate towards yourself when things go wrong, celebrate what goes well, and remind yourself that you deserve success.

REFLECTIVE EXAMPLE

I'm feeling good today! I slept well last night and woke up to sunshine, the perfect beginning of the day. While I was dozing, I ran through my mind all the nice things that happened yesterday. Then I planned my day and told myself it would all go well: three patients in the morning, a quick lunch, desk work and then walk to the school to collect my kids rather than take the car. I reminded myself that my aim for the day was to help my patients, do some good work, and boost my confidence with as many ☺ awards (smiley face awards) as I could!

9.00am: phone call from patient X wanting an appointment for today.

9.30am: my first patient arrived late, but I was in the flow and I negotiated that she should have a slightly shorter treatment session because she was late.

☺ My first smile today for negotiating.

10.00am: the patient left and I had time to write up my notes and get a cup of tea.

☺ My second smile today for writing up notes between all my patients.

10.15am–11.00am: second patient. Everything went well.

11.15am–12.00pm: third patient. This is the patient who talks all the time about her wayward son. For the first time, I felt I could gently interrupt her, and steer her into telling me useful information. To my surprise, she wasn't in the least offended about being interrupted. I felt I could work well after that, and for the first time with this patient I finished on time. What a breakthrough!

☺ My third smile today for setting the boundaries and finishing on time.

12.00pm–1.30pm: I was so, so tempted to have lunch at my desk, but instead I made a sandwich and had it in the garden in the sunshine. While I was sitting there I realized that I needed to put the desk work into two piles, the essential/urgent work and the non-essential. It was like a light bulb came on, and to be honest if I'd started the desk work while eating lunch I wouldn't have thought of it. I was able to get through all of the essential pile after lunch.

☺ My fourth smile today for taking the time out for lunch (and having that idea).

1.45pm–2.30pm: My final patient, the old chap who phoned up this morning. He was so grateful, I felt pleased I'd managed to fit him in.

2.45pm: Left the house to collect the kids from school.

☺ My fifth smile today for not taking the car and getting some exercise. Well done me.

Sum total = ☺ ☺ ☺ ☺ ☺ five smiley face awards for today!

EXERCISE: VISUALIZING A GOOD-FEELING PRACTICE

If you wish you can get someone else to read this out slowly to you. Sit in a comfortable and quiet room, cross-legged or with both feet on the floor, your hands relaxed, and your eyes closed. Become aware of your breathing and allow yourself to breathe naturally for a few minutes.

Be aware of any sounds around you in the room, but try to keep your mind free of thoughts. Every time your mind wanders bring it back to the present. After a few minutes of breathing naturally, take a few deep breaths, and as you breathe out, consciously relax your face and neck muscles with the out-breath. Return to normal breathing.

Imagine it is Christmas, and all of your patients have written you a Christmas card. Each card has a short, heartfelt and positive appreciation of your work written inside.

Hold the bundle of cards in your hands and accept that the thanks and appreciation expressed are all for you.

Consider your feelings on receiving these cards. Do you feel excitement, cheerfulness, satisfaction or improved self-confidence? Imagine the smile on your face, imagine your heart swelling with exhilaration, the feeling of being in the flow, the feeling that all is well. How do you express yourself physically when everything is going your way? Do you jump up and down, sing, dance or laugh? Could you draw or paint that feeling? Hold onto that good feeling for as long as possible.

Allow yourself to gently come back to the present, and when you're ready make a few notes to yourself about that good feeling you felt in the visualization. That is what you want to feel about your practice. You don't need to think in terms of how much and how many. Just visualize the good feelings.

EXERCISE: ACKNOWLEDGE YOUR STRENGTHS

Write a long boasting list of the wealth of experiences, values and qualities that you bring to your profession as a practitioner. You will have your official qualification such as your graduation certificate, but what else do you bring to your practice? This is the opportunity to acknowledge your strengths in terms of your character and personality as well as your skills, knowledge and experience.

EXERCISE: LIST THE POSITIVE ASPECTS

For a week or more, keep a notebook by the side of your bed and every evening write a list of at least six things that went well for you today. These can be things that you initiated, or that other people said to you or did for you, but they all need to be positive things that made you feel good. For example, someone made you smile, you did half an hour of really good work with a difficult patient, you remembered to make *that* phone call, a patient shook your hand to say thank you or you made time to have a healthy lunch.

The difference between the boasting list and the list of positive aspects is that the boasting list is all about your achievements and the list of positive aspects is about what has happened to you, both through what you did and what other people did.

EXERCISE: SELF-COMPASSION

Think of three different occasions in the last few months where you have made a mistake, but learned something from it – such as going out on a windy day without a coat and getting rained on. You learned to take your coat for the rest of the week. Or you were very rude to a cold-caller on the phone, and a week later someone was rude to you on the phone. Review each of these occasions through the eyes of self-compassion. This means that you should be understanding and kind to yourself so that you can feel comfortable and open to learning from them.

For example: 'I don't like the way I was rude to that telesales person, but I can see that it came from my frustration when I was trying to do too much at once. I'm usually calm and polite when I answer my phone. I'm feeling sorry about it now but feeling guilty won't change the past. I'm not the first or the last person to vent my anger on the phone, and I'll be more aware of my behaviour in future. I know what it feels like to be on the receiving end of such rudeness. I got back what I gave out, which seems to be what the law of attraction is about. That's okay, I've learned from it. The next time I get a telesales call I will remember they are just doing their job and I'll treat them with kindness.'

Chapter 2

BEFORE THE PATIENT ARRIVES

Being a patient is just a role, it's not a chronic condition. It is one half of the practitioner–patient relationship and outside of this the person has many areas of their life in which they are fully autonomous and independent. When we talk about someone as a patient, we mean that they have entered into a relationship with a health practitioner, on the understanding that the practitioner will try to heal the discomfort (the dis-ease) or at least remove the symptoms. Maybe in calling them 'patient' we are asking them to be patient with us, the practitioners.

It is worth asking yourself what the patient's wants, hopes and needs are in coming to an alternative practitioner. Many adults are in a position to choose what practitioner they visit, and most start with a visit to their general practitioner. By the time they arrive at the clinic of the alternative practitioner, many will have built up a complex history of their symptoms, their personal analysis of what is happening, the doctor's diagnosis and any medication they are currently taking. Their hopes and needs on entering this new patient–practitioner relationship, might vary considerably, depending upon this history.

It is easy to see what patients don't want: to be judged, blamed, infantilized or treated as a case number. Sometimes it is more difficult to see what the patient does want. As a practitioner, we might fantasize about the cooperative, intelligent and knowledgeable patient who is a pleasure to talk to and easy to treat, but not everyone is going to be like this. Some people arrive hoping for a practitioner who has both the practical expertise and the compassionate, spiritual abilities of the healer or shaman. Others are looking for the supportive, caring qualities of the archetypal nurturing parent; or someone to take responsibility and just tell them what to do. Some people arrive with a negative attitude and low expectations, following their experiences with practitioners who have no skills of rapport. Yet others are looking for someone to collude with, a partnership that is safe and does not challenge the status quo.

Most people will do a careful assessment of available practitioners in order to choose one they can develop a good working relationship with. This assessment process is done both consciously and unconsciously, using logical reasoning (this practitioner is more expensive/local than that one) and tuning into non-verbal signals (this one feels right). Even when asking for a referral from a friend, they will take note of the warmth and enthusiasm shown, as well as the content of the answer. If they phone up to make enquiries, the practitioner's tone of voice, pace of the answer, and the interest expressed all contribute towards their final decision. In searching the Internet, even more subtle clues are picked up from the visual impact of the website, the photograph of the practitioner and the clarity of the content. The potential patient might be unaware of how much they are intuitively assessing each practitioner, but they will often follow their gut reaction or feeling about who will suit them best.

If you have doubts about this, reflect for a few minutes about how quickly you made up your mind about any new doctor, dentist or alternative practitioner that you have visited. You might have overridden your initial instinctive reaction for the sake of expediency, and you might concede that your practitioner was having an off day when you first met them, but often you will trust your first reaction.

I know that when I'm looking for a new practitioner, I will look for someone who has appropriate experience and good knowledge in their speciality; *and* some of the nurturing qualities such as empathy, approachability, trustworthiness, respect, support, genuineness, understanding, gentleness or compassion. I suggest that most patients are looking for the same thing. The nurturing qualities are the higher values or more spiritual qualities that inform the practitioner's attitude towards the patient. Without them the practitioner appears to be a scientist with no bedside manner. With these higher values there is compassion, nourishment and healing (see Figure 2.1). I have not attempted to list all of these values; it is a long list and it continues to expand.

When I needed some specialist dental treatment, my dentist recommended a local dental hospital where I was interviewed by one practitioner and a month later given the treatment by a different one. I am not at my ease in a dental chair and didn't feel ready to open my mouth until I had found out what sort of person would be working on my teeth. But to my relief, he had a gentle voice, introduced himself and his assistant, gave me eye contact and explained carefully what he planned to do. I was able to relax, not because of his explanation as such, but because I felt respected and spoken to as an equal. He continued explaining the process as he worked so that I was able to take more of an outsider's view of what was happening and detach from my own discomfort. When he finished the procedure, he gave instructions about food intake for the next 24 hours and asked me if I had any questions.

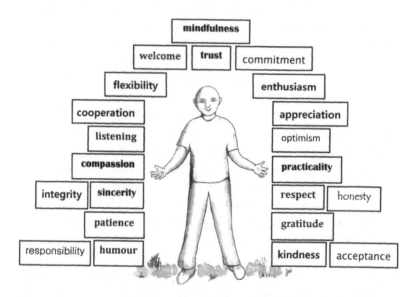

FIGURE 2.1: CHOOSE TO BE AN OPEN-HEARTED PRACTITIONER

My dentist chose this hospital because of their expertise and experience. When I got there I found respect alongside understanding, gentleness and compassion. The specialist must have seen hundreds of patients with similar conditions, but taking a few minutes to relate to me as a person rather than as a patient made a huge difference to my experience.

PERSONAL PREPARATION

An outsider might imagine that all a student practitioner needs to do in order to see patients, would be to study their particular therapy until they have both the knowledge and skills to perform it. The specialist knowledge can be found in books or on the Internet, while the skills come from repeated practice. I suggest there are three other tools that the practitioner needs to have in order to be successful (see Box 2.1). One of these is to fully understand and be able to put into practice your code of ethics. If you do not belong to an association that has its own code of ethics or do not have one for any other reason, you should research into what is generally understood to be ethical behaviour (see Chapter 10).

BOX 2.1 THE PRACTITIONER IS READY FOR PATIENTS WHEN THEY HAVE...

- intellectual knowledge of the therapy
- practical skills of the therapy
- knowledge of their code of ethics
- understanding of the practitioner–patient relationship
- self-understanding and commitment to self-development.

The next area is to have some understanding of the practitioner–patient dynamic. Alternative practitioners understand and relish the thought that everyone is different and everyone has their own individual characteristics. This provides for an infinite variety of cases to treat, but also creates some interesting variations on the practitioner–patient relationship. Some of these will open you up to new ideas and new possibilities, while others will break your boundaries and disturb you. If you have some reference points to help you understand what's going on, then you can analyse what has happened and either renegotiate with this patient or be more prepared for future patients (see Chapter 3).

Finally and most importantly, the practitioner needs self-knowledge and a commitment to self-development. If you understand yourself, and you know where your prejudices lie and what triggers your emotional reactions, you will be more neutral and compassionate with your patients. Much as we would like to imagine that we don't bring ourselves into the consulting room when we are practitioners, we cannot be neutral simply by wanting to be so. Take a few minutes to remember the person from your childhood who irritated you the most – even if it was done for good reasons, like your mother nagging you to study harder. Then imagine how you would react if your patient had a personality very similar to this irritating person.

Keeping with the same example, you either have to refuse to see all patients who remind you of your childhood bully, or you have to release your inner prejudice against people with that particular attitude and tone of voice. If you see the patient while you are carrying your prejudice from the past, you won't be able to help them. If you decide to release your prejudice, it might take some time while you learn how to forgive the other person. Sometimes it's helpful to understand your childhood from that other person's point of view.

Patients can arrive who have different personal values from you that might have come from their education, their experience, their social group, their religious community or their personal ethics. If these start to concern you, then you are no longer the neutral practitioner. I remember one patient who was talking about her 11-year-old son with pride, because he would buy a toy from a large toyshop, play with it for a week, then carefully repackage it and take it back, to exchange it for another one. He had been doing this for months. This completely went against my own values, and my shock at her pride in and complicity with her son stopped me in my tracks. I had to pretend to re-read my notes in order to collect myself and come back into case-taking mode.

I have written a lot about self-reflection in my book *Transformation through Journal Writing* (Wood 2012). I find there is immense value in keeping a journal, in which you can record issues as they come up for you, and start to explore them (see Chapter 13). The journal becomes a record that can be re-read at any time, notifying you when the same issues repeat themselves in different forms. This inner work on yourself can begin at any stage, while you are a student or as a mature practitioner. You just need to be alert to your own inner reactions to experiences and be willing to do the self-development.

As you do the work on yourself, you begin to let go of some of the issues you have been trailing behind you since childhood, and you learn to listen to your patient's stories without surprise, prejudice or judgement. For me, after meeting the proud mother whose son exchanged toys, I didn't waste time chastising myself for being prejudiced, or blaming her for being immoral. I wanted to reach the place where I could feel compassion for her as a patient, regardless of her money values. I spent some time making a list of what I do that might shock or surprise her, as she had shocked me. Then I looked at what I could appreciate about her. The next time we met I could look at her with more compassion, accepting that we are all different and may not have the same values.

You will see that I have given reflective journal examples at the end of each chapter, to show you a variety of issues and different ways of reflecting. There are also various exercises that might trigger your own self-reflection.

THE PATIENT'S FIRST CONTACT

Each new patient is a challenge that can be exciting and invigorating for the practitioner – or could drag you out of your depth with complicated emotional or physical pathology. It is worth preparing before the patient comes.

If you're busy as a practitioner you might have a receptionist, but if you answer all phone calls, texts and e-mails yourself it is to your advantage. It gives you the opportunity to engage with the potential patient for a few moments and try to make a good impression. You can inform and explain about your therapy while consciously using communication skills like a reassuring tone of voice, asking how much they already know, sympathizing – and holding a boundary if they start to talk about their symptoms. A similar process happens with e-mail, although it is more limited and more difficult to judge their emotions.

Answering phone enquiries is something that can (and should!) be practised by student practitioners in role-play. At first it appears to be easy because they are trained to be specialists in their subject, but when I have asked students to do this in role-play, they often stumble and come to a halt. Most of them find it very difficult to explain their therapy in an accessible way, with limited time and to a person that they cannot see. It requires pre-planning with pen and paper, rehearsal time in role-play, and feedback from the role-play partner. Eventually you will develop the skill of an experienced telesales person, giving out information in easily digestible quantities, engaging the other in conversation and offering to mail out further information.

After the phone call, if the appointment has been made, you can jot down your first impressions. It is surprising how much information can be picked up during a five-minute phone call, including the tone of voice, energy, confidence and knowledge level of the caller. This is not to say that first impressions are always correct, but this early information, when added to the rest of the consultation, will help to build up an overall picture of the patient. For many practitioners, the consultation starts before the patient arrives.

A newly graduated practitioner that I was supervising told me about a patient who had phoned him for an appointment. The patient's first words were to express dissatisfaction with her previous practitioner. Then she began talking about her symptoms which were so numerous that the practitioner felt he should be taking notes; and this was before they had even booked a first appointment. He felt uneasy about her, and on discussion he realized this came from her relish in describing her symptoms.

The issues with a phone call like this are twofold. If a potential patient starts off the phone call with grumbling about the previous practitioner, there is a high possibility they will be dissatisfied with the next one, which could be you. The other issue is the patient's apparent enjoyment of talking about her symptoms. It sounded as if she had a big investment in being ill, and enjoyed being in a victim role. This would probably be a quite difficult case to treat.

Another practitioner might want to take on this case as a welcome challenge, even with the risks attached of hypochondria and a grumbling patient. But the practitioner who received this phone call didn't think he had enough experience to deal with such a long-term patient. He decided that even though there were appointments available, he would be out of his depth with this patient, and he phoned her back to say sorry, he didn't think he could help her.

PREPARING THE CONSULTING ROOM

Your consulting room is much more than an office; it contributes its own energy towards the healing connection between practitioner and patient. Consulting rooms in hospitals and health centres are often designed with efficiency, hygiene or practicality in mind, giving doctors or nurses little choice about their environment. The alternative practitioner has more choice over the appearance, comfort and energy of the room. A practitioner writes:

> I learned that when I'm looking for somewhere to work away from home, I should make it a good place. It sounds obvious but it isn't, my first clinic space was completely soulless, cold and empty...

on the bright side it was cheap. But it was never going to attract patients. I sat there for three days each week growing increasingly dispirited with only the occasional patient. It was an out-of-the-way place and lonely. I reflected on my experience and saw that the clinic's lack of positive energy would not draw people seeking help for their own poor state.

I decided to find somewhere that was already a vibrant, healing space. My practice is now in a chiropractic clinic with every type of therapist working there. It already has like-minded practitioners and patients coming to see them. I found that it is far better to have fewer affordable hours and pay more, than lots of access to somewhere out of the way and cheap.

(Kathryn Walker in private correspondence with
Jane Wood, reproduced with permission)

If you're practising from home, you can probably choose your own colours, furnishings, positioning of furniture, and you can regulate the temperature and air flow of the clinic room. If you're practising in a rented clinic you might have control over some of these. They are all a form of non-verbal communication that can contribute to or detract from your patient's emotional or physical comfort. Have a look around your clinic room and consider the body language of the furniture. Does it appear open and welcoming or clinical and uncomfortable? If the room is small, are you sitting too close to each other and feeling cramped or intimidated? Are you a practitioner that sits behind a desk? This can create a physical and emotional barrier which is doubled if you're typing into a computer as well.

A colleague of mine has had to move house in the same area several times over a few years and she always works from home. She maintains exactly the same furniture, books and arrangements in each new clinic room, so that all of her patients feel comfortable in a familiar environment.

Try sitting in the patient's chair and check their sightlines towards where you would be sitting. Is the general impression one of orderliness or untidiness – and which would be more comfortable for most patients? If the patient is to lie upon a treatment couch, what are they looking up towards? Make sure you brush away all the old spider's webs.

Consider what impact the colours of the clinic room might have on the patient. Should they be warm, welcoming colours or cool, calming colours? Do you want all of your text books on display, giving the non-verbal message that you have studied a lot?

If you are planning to see children as part of your practice, you need to make the clinic room child-safe, and have a box of suitable toys. Personally I lose concentration if there are toys with electronic sound effects or music, so these are banned from my consulting room. I have a basket full of small cars, a selection of dinosaurs and other animals, a doll's house peopled by cute, clothed animals. There are a few baby toys and the standard pencils and paper as well.

JUST BEFORE THE PATIENT ARRIVES

If you have time, take ten minutes before your patient comes to quieten your mind and mentally prepare. Perhaps 'mentally prepare' are the wrong words. Glance around the room to check it is tidy, making sure that the previous person's imprint has been shaken out of the cushions and their notes have been put away. Then sit in your usual chair, close your eyes and focus on your breathing, allowing yourself to slow down and open your heart to the person who is on their way. You could do the three-minute or the one-minute meditation described in Chapter 5.

For some practitioners the day starts with taking their children to school and then racing back to make sure that their clinic room and the bathroom are clean and tidy, before the first patient arrives. Running on such a tight time schedule means that you have to clear your desk the night before as well as do any other preparations. I don't recommend this as an ideal way of working, but it can be the reality for many parents.

Some practitioners like to do a small ritual before seeing patients, to focus themselves inwards on their work and put aside personal issues. These rituals might be changing into smart clothes, lighting a candle, putting on an overall, watering the plants or reading a few lines of something uplifting. If you find that you are very sensitive to the influence of your patients, you might need to do a protection ritual before seeing anyone. You could quietly visualize a bubble of white or coloured light that completely surrounds you and holds you safe; or draw three large hula hoops in the air, one around your waist, one front to back, and one side to side (see Chapter 12's section 'Separating from the patient').

After the patient leaves, you need at least five or ten minutes (preferably 15) to clear the clinic room and attend to any of your personal needs such as hunger, thirst or going to the bathroom. You should take time to clear your mind of the previous patient before seeing the next one. Different practitioners achieve this in different ways. Sometimes the ritual of tidying up is enough, such as filing the notes or completed questionnaire, stripping off the paper sheeting from the treatment couch or putting away the toys. At other times it is helpful to open the window or the door, wash your hands or do some breathing exercises. If the case has been a particularly emotional or traumatic one, you can light an incense stick and carry it around the room close to the walls; spray around the room with a dedicated clearing spray or sound a ringing bowl or bell in the room – providing you don't startle a patient in the waiting room.

BE PREPARED

If you prepare yourself and your clinic room before the patient comes, then you can be totally present and mindful when you're with them. If you're not prepared, you might spend the first part of the consultation listening to your inner voices rather than tending to your patient.

Being an alternative practitioner brings with it the huge privilege of getting to know your patients and hearing their stories. Some patients you will get to know on a deeper, more intimate level than their families and loved ones know them. Other patients will teach you to know yourself on a deeper level than you had ever imagined. Prepare yourself as much as is reasonable, remind yourself that everyone is different and greet each patient with an open mind.

▊ REFLECTIVE EXAMPLE

A couple of days ago a receptionist at the opticians phoned me up to say they were planning to turn two of the back rooms of the shop into therapy rooms, and would I be interested in working there. I have to admit I was flattered. I've never been headhunted before. Today I went to have a look at the rooms, and discuss terms and conditions. The rent is fairly high, so I said I would probably start with one morning every two weeks and build it up from there. But I need to think through everything more carefully before I sign anything.

The advantages of joining the clinic are...

A receptionist to book in my patients, a shop front on the High Street, a proper sign in the window listing all the different therapies, working in a multi-therapy practice (which I have always wanted to do), being able to choose how many hours I will do, and hopefully when it opens as an alternative clinic we can arrange for a local newspaper to do an article on it.

The disadvantages are...

It's expensive, I would still have to do my own advertising, and I would have to carry my case notes and other equipment whenever I go there. The greatest disadvantage and the one that is worrying me, is that the rooms are small, overheated and have no windows. The optician has had the walls painted grey and had grey carpets put down. He was pleased with this colour, which he said was neutral, but to me it looked dull and slightly depressing. It's a sort of hospital colour, and gives me a bad feeling. I'm not the sort of person who gets claustrophobic, but my guess is that some (many?) of my patients really won't like these clinic rooms.

What should I do?

There do seem to be a lot of advantages, but my instinct tells me that it is just not going to suit anyone who is sensitive to atmospheres. An optician needs a room with no window, but all the rest of us need daylight and oxygen to put our patients at ease. My choices are: try it out for 3–6 months or simply turn it down. Why am I hesitating? Because another practitioner might take it and make a success of it and then I will regret my decision. Do I want to be a dog in the manger, taking on a clinic room that I don't want, just to prevent someone else getting it? No, that would be crazy.

Okay, I've decided...

I will turn it down, and try not to think about it any more. No regrets! Instead I will visualize a better clinic coming my way, with bigger brighter rooms and a friendly receptionist.

EXERCISE: PRACTISE A TELEPHONE ENQUIRY

Write down and memorize a two- or three-minute introduction to your therapy. This needs to be both simple and honest. Then try it out with a family member, friend or classmate who is willing to role-play a prospective patient phoning up to make enquiries. Make sure you do not have eye contact with your role-play partner, sitting back to back or in a different room. Make a note of anything you stumbled over, have a rethink about what you could have said, and then try again with another role-play. These are valuable rehearsals, allowing you to practise until you're comfortable with phone enquiries.

EXERCISE: MINDFULLY ASSESS YOUR CLINIC ROOM

Sit alone in the clinic room, in either the patient's chair or your practitioner's chair. Sit with both feet on the floor, and relax your neck and shoulders while keeping your head upright. Let the seat take your weight. Listen to your breathing and try to feel present in the room, just listening to the sounds around you, feeling the temperature of the air, noticing any smell. If you find yourself thinking of something else, just quietly come back into your awareness of the room again. Do this for three to five minutes and then gently open your eyes.

Remaining quietly in your chair, try to feel the atmosphere of your clinic room. Is it warm, comfortable, safe, inviting or peaceful? Or is it cold, stiff, demanding or clashing? I suggest that you start with the overall feeling then consider the individual senses. What does your clinic room feel like? For example, visually bright or contrasting colours are fun and vibrant, but may not give messages of trust and empathy. Foliage plants or a window that looks out onto greenery might be more relaxing, but plants that are dusty or needing water might give another message. If there is a window, can other people look in?

Notice whether there are any distractions in the room and decide whether this is what you want or not. A busy pattern or a beautiful picture might demand the patient's attention, distracting them from the acupuncturist's needles – or preventing them from explaining themselves properly to the homeopath. Outside noise can be irritating and there needs to be adequate insulation to prevent the patient's words being overheard. Can you open a window to get fresh air without losing privacy? The cleanliness of the floor or feel of seating fabrics can invite or repel and a room that is too cold or too dark might make the patient tense.

Once you have made your assessment, decide if there's anything you want to improve. What changes can be made without causing too much expense or upheaval?

EXERCISE: SELF-REFLECTION

Think back to your best experience as a patient with a practitioner. Make a list of what that practitioner did to make you award them top marks. Was it what they said, their attitude, their understanding of your case or anything else? Did they have any of the nurturing qualities, such as kindness, honesty, genuineness and so on? You might want to contrast this with your worst experience as a patient.

What ideas can you borrow from your top-marks practitioner? Try to think of some changes that you could introduce into your time with the patient that would improve their experience when they come to your clinic?

Chapter 3

RELATIONSHIP MODELS IN THE CONSULTING ROOM

In western medicine the roles used to be clear: the doctor made the decisions because he (rarely she) had the knowledge and experience, and the patient cooperated by doing what they were told. This follows a paternalistic model, similar to that of the teacher–student or lawyer–client relationships. One person holds all the power and the other one is perceived to lack knowledge, understanding, experience or power. It's an attitude that was (and is) perpetuated by many different professionals through the use of technical language and jargon. It is expressed in the old joke about a man who goes to the doctor with an ear infection and comes home with a diagnosis of *otitis media* – which is simply the Latin name for a middle ear infection.

PATERNALISM AND MUTUALITY: TWO DIFFERENT MODELS

Paternalism has its advantages. It gives the doctor or practitioner a great deal of control over the interview process as well as the prescription, so consultations are kept to time. In *Skills for Communicating with Patients*, Silverman, Kurtz and Draper (2005) suggest that the paternalist model might suit people who are seriously ill or vulnerable, and might be the preference of the elderly or the less well-educated. In these cases, the patient may choose to be passive and not take an active part in the consultation or decision-making process (p.178). Silverman *et al.* (2005) reference a study where:

> Physicians deliberately used highly technical language to control communication and to limit patient questions – such behaviour occurred twice as often when doctors were under pressure of time. (p.143)

Another argument for using the paternalistic model is that illness causes so much negative emotion that it prevents rational communication – or that illness makes the patient passive and dependent (although it's open to debate whether it's the illness or the doctor that makes them passive). Paternalism helps the doctor maintain clinical detachment and defend against emotional contamination from the patient:

> In traditional medical education, much is made of the need to protect ourselves from the powerful emotions of medical practice where feelings are painful for both patient and doctor. Impassive objectivity is recommended as a coping mechanism. (Silverman *et al.* 2005, p.120)

The disadvantages of the paternalistic model are that it can give the doctor too much of a sense of their own power, so that they forget to be compassionate. It forces the patient into a passive role where they are expected to be compliant, do what they're told like a child, and not ask any intelligent questions. This can leave the patient in a state of frustration or indignation because they were not listened to and don't feel understood. The same happens when the consultation is too short to get to the heart of the matter.

A different model is that of mutuality, where there is cooperation between doctor and patient. This means the interview contains more interaction between them and the patient is included in the decision-making process. Patients are asked for their preferences and the doctor or practitioner openly discusses their knowledge and opinions, until they reach a mutually negotiated plan. With Internet searches available, many patients are reasonably well-informed about their illness and some are highly knowledgeable. Doctors themselves are more able to share information either verbally or through printing off fact-sheets. Research has shown that when the patient is involved in the decision-making, they are much more likely to finish the treatment recommended by the doctor. In turn, this means less wastage of time, resources and money:

> Increasingly, health professionals are moving away from the use of the word 'compliance' altogether, with its overtones of passivity, obedience and 'following doctor's orders.' (Silverman *et al.* 2005, p.181)

Most alternative practitioners prefer to use the mutuality model. They approach the patient on a human level and use a cooperative interview process, followed by a negotiated treatment plan. There is no expectation that the patient is too weak, passive or dependent to think for themselves, but occasionally they may choose to hand over the decision-making to the practitioner. The advantages of cooperation are many: it shows respect for the patient's autonomy, it builds up trust, it shares the responsibility and it treats every patient as an individual requiring their own treatment plan. The more the patient is involved, the more likely they are to return, which gives the practitioner a greater chance to heal them. The practitioner still holds much of the power because of their knowledge and experience, but as Su Fox (2008) writing in *Relating to Clients: The Therapeutic Relationship for Complementary Therapists*, points out it can be used to empower the patient:

> We have chosen, by virtue of being complementary therapists, to help others and with that decision comes power, not in the sense that the word is often understood, but in the sense that we are in a position to facilitate healing. (p.111)

Alternative practitioners are less wary than doctors about witnessing the patient's emotions. In over 20 years working as a homeopath, I would say up to half of my patients would cry at some time or other. As well as being a release for the patient, it frequently helped me highlight the key issues for the patient that needed to be healed. I kept a big box of tissues on the desk and felt deep compassion. I learned to give the patient time to cry. If I did feel a strong emotion after hearing a patient's story that stayed with me afterwards, I took the time to process it through supervision or self-reflection.

Alternative therapy sessions can be over an hour long, so the practitioner does not need to control the conversation because of time restrictions. The longer interview allows the patient time to relax and explain themselves on a deeper level. However, the disadvantage of a longer interview is that the patient has the time to start enacting, rather than just describing their emotional pathology and the practitioner can get caught up in this.

From the patient's point of view, this is not conscious or deliberate. They might be hoping for an adult conversation with a mutually agreed outcome, without realizing that they bring with them their previous experiences of different practitioner–patient relationships. This might be the patient who has previous experience of feeling overpowered by the status or the arrogance of a health professional

– or even that of a parent or carer – which they can carry into the next patient–practitioner relationship. They might subconsciously play out the relationship patterns that they are used to, by falling into accustomed roles. The practitioner can easily get drawn into playing the opposite and balancing role, like a couple of children on a seesaw. This distorts the relationship and can confuse both case-taking and the subsequent treatment. If the practitioner notices these subconscious patterns being played out, they can choose to consciously step off the seesaw (see Figure 3.1).

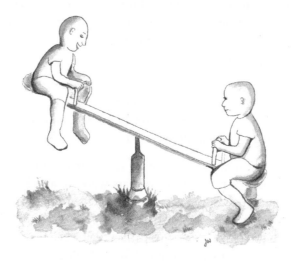

FIGURE 3.1: GET OFF THE SEESAW OF POWER

Examples of these subconscious patterns are in the following models.

THE DRAMA TRIANGLE

This was identified by Karpman (1968) and is a shorthand way of describing the dynamics of a temporary relationship between two or three people. There are three characters in the Drama Triangle: the Victim, the Rescuer and the Persecutor. These are psychological stances and nothing to do with genuine hardship, belonging to the emergency services or even litigious bullies. Anyone can take any role at any time. The Persecutor feels they need to control or bully the other person, maybe from an inner insecurity, or maybe because they simply enjoy conflict. This behaviour can give them a sense of power or superiority. They can be angry and aggressive and can have a clear image of right and wrong. The Victim is the one who suffers from the bully and appears to be the weakest character in the game because they discount their own power. They appear to be helpless and complaining and generally enjoy other people taking care of them. They might be passively obstinate about not taking responsibility, and this obstinacy gives them back a measure of power. The third role is that of Rescuer who likes to look after and care for others, in particular the Victim. It gives them meaning in their lives and makes them feel needed. Rescuing can give them a sense of superiority. Generally they are patient, responsible and kind. A long-term Rescuer might become dependent upon having someone to rescue and could have an investment in preventing the Victim from flourishing.

There are several ways that this could play out within the practitioner–patient relationship. A common one observed by alternative practitioners is when the patient takes the role of Victim. As they tell their history, they focus on their suffering (the disease becomes the Persecutor) or their previous treatment by the medical profession (the medical profession are seen as the Persecutor) or other alternative practitioners (the previous practitioners are Persecutors). This can invoke the current practitioner's need to be a Rescuer. The practitioner hopes to be the one person who can successfully help this patient. So eager are they to rescue this patient that they might give the patient extra time either through a longer appointment, phone calls after hours or studying the case at the weekend. They might do the patient small favours, seeking to make them feel better or make their lives easier.

Boundaries begin to falter and the patient becomes dependent and loses any reason to take responsibility for themselves. Both keep acting out their role, maintaining the status quo between sick victim and rescuing practitioner. Eventually, the practitioner might feel exhausted and somewhat claustrophobic, and risk becoming the new Persecutor.

Less common is when the patient takes the role of Rescuer, noticing the practitioner's weaknesses and offering to help. All patients are capable of noticing practitioner's strengths and weaknesses, but the Rescuer wants to become involved, in order to feel good. It is as if the patient is pushing the practitioner into Victim mode. Examples would be the patient who offers to take letters to the post or walk the dog for the practitioner. This behaviour, which would be welcome from a friend, changes the practitioner–patient relationship.

Finally the patient can take the role of Persecutor, bullying the practitioner into working harder or longer on their case. The bullying can be subtle, expressed through body language and facial expression, as well as overtly questioning the working agreement or even the therapy itself. This could be the patient who comes to the homeopath, saying, 'I don't believe in homeopathy, but my partner persuaded me to come.' The practitioner starts to feel uncomfortable, as they are being challenged to prove something, and frequently they do work harder, only to feel resentful and victimized. If the practitioner feels like a Victim, they will probably talk through the case with a colleague or supervisor, in the hope that someone will Rescue them. In this instance, rescue might take the form of commiseration and suggestions about how to deal with the challenging patient.

For many practitioners, their favourite role is that of Rescuer, which is probably a role they have been performing since childhood. They feel good when looking after and caring for others and it gives them meaning in their life. It is what draws them to join the caring professions. The risk is that they could lose their boundaries with patients, do too much and become burnt out. A practitioner in the Rescuer mode is in danger of disempowering themselves in order to empower the patient.

The Drama Triangle is often played out in the consulting room. A mother and teenage daughter came to my clinic for the first time. They had obviously had an argument in the car and both arrived with tight, angry faces and stiff body language. The mother was the first to recover herself, and politely went through all the preliminaries with me even though it was her daughter who was the patient. The daughter had eczema and the mother described herself sympathetically conceding to her daughter's requests for clothes, accessories and piercings. The problem was that the girl had become very tempestuous over the last few years. The mother described her daughter as a bully at home and clearly presented herself as a Victim, persecuted by the 14-year-old who sat glowering next to her. I could see that I was being invited to rescue the mother, and reason with the girl. Instead I chose to speak directly to the girl and ask her opinion.

Hesitant at first, the girl began telling her side of the story, revealing how she felt persecuted by the eczema, persecuted by a few classmates who teased her and persecuted by her mother. The mother found it difficult to sit still and listen to this, because she hated the image of herself cast as Persecutor. She kept interrupting to deny what her daughter was saying, to the point when I found myself answering her back, taking the girl's side. Having avoided rescuing the mother, I was now rescuing the daughter. Both of them saw themselves as victim, with the other one as persecutor, and it was such a strong dynamic that frequently the father took one side or the other as Rescuer. It was unsurprising that I got pulled into it as well.

I was lucky to spot this while it was happening. I had to move fast before the mother could build up resentment for my disloyalty. After all, she was paying for the consultation. I hastily offered the mother a compliment on her input and suggested that it would be easier for me if I interviewed them separately, starting with the daughter.

TRANSFERENCE AND COUNTERTRANSFERENCE

Transference is a term used when someone unconsciously refers back to their relationship with their parents or other people who influenced them, and assumes the current relationship with its attendant emotions will be the same. Patients can unknowingly and inappropriately transfer feelings from a past relationship onto the current practitioner. They might expect the new practitioner to be aloof and unapproachable, or sympathetic and friendly like the previous one. They might have unspoken expectations of the practitioner that are completely outside of the working agreement. For example, they might expect to socialize with the practitioner, or they expect them to return phone calls immediately whatever the time of day or night. In this last example, the patient might be referring back to one of their parents whose unconditional love and anxiety had them in constant contact.

Countertransference is a term used for the practitioner's unconscious feelings towards the patient, either in reply to the transference, or spontaneously arising. Sometimes your inner judge (see 'The inner judge and the inner justifier' section later in this chapter) takes time off from criticizing you, and turns to criticize other people, perhaps the patient. You might witness this, when you start thinking that your patient 'should' behave in a certain way.

THE THREE EGO STATES

The three ego states were defined by Berne (1961). They are a 'state of being or experience which involves our thinking, feeling, and behaving' (Lapworth and Stills 2011, p.25). The ego states occur regardless of the person's actual age. The Child ego state comes directly from childhood experience stored in the unconscious and influences moods or behaviour in the present. It can be expressed as either the free Child who is spontaneous and playful or the compensated Child whose behaviour is set in a fixed pattern that goes back to childhood. Examples of the compensated Child would be compliance or resistance when these are automatic behaviours rather than appropriate ones.

The Parent ego state is built up from childhood memories of parents and parental figures, stored in the unconscious and directing current behaviour, thoughts or feelings. When this ego state is present, the person could find themselves unexpectedly repeating long forgotten behaviours or words from their past. The Parent ego state can be expressed as either nurturing or criticizing. Finally, the Adult ego state is in direct relation to the current reality, with no historical interference. It is present, balanced and reacts appropriately.

Each ego state is displayed when a person joins in a temporary or long-term relationship with someone else, such as the practitioner–patient relationship. Any combination of the three roles is possible for each relationship. Common patterns are a comfortable dynamic with both of them in Adult role; or an uncomfortable relationship with one of them as Parent and the other one as Child. (There are further more complex patterns than the ones described here.)

There are many ways that this could play out in the practitioner–patient relationship. The patient can appear in Child mode, usually the compensated Child wanting to be a 'good' patient, prompting the practitioner to become the nurturing Parent. Another version of the compensated Child might be the closed down patient who finds it difficult to describe their symptoms – which could produce in the practitioner a critical Parent who becomes impatient and irritable. A sad or weeping patient can trigger in the practitioner either a nurturing Parent or a critical Parent, according to their own patterns and attitudes.

The practitioner who decides on personal values and protocols in clinic above and beyond what is recommended in their code of ethics, is probably reacting to their inner critical Parent. ('You ought to write up your notes every evening.') The practitioner who constantly seeks help with their cases, can be reacting to their inner compensated Child. ('If I make mistakes, I'll get told off so I'll get others to help.')

A practitioner came to me for supervision because she was having confidence issues over a patient. The patient was older than her, considerably wealthier and she had specifically chosen the practitioner because they were of the same religion. This had happened before with the practitioner and she usually felt fine about it. But this particular woman was more orthodox than the practitioner, higher up the social hierarchy, and had a superior manner. She kept mentioning religious observances that she felt the practitioner should participate in. The practitioner felt unable to stand up to her and believed she ought to do as the other suggested. Her Child ego was full of awe for her patient's strong, critical Parent and on that level she was ready to comply immediately. On another level, she recognized this was unreasonable and had come to supervision to discuss it.

THE INNER JUDGE AND THE INNER JUSTIFIER

Elsewhere I have written (Wood 2012) how we all carry an inner judge and an inner justifier. The inner judge I equate with the Parent ego state in critical mode, and the inner justifier I equate with the Child ego state in defensive or compensated mode. The inner judge has a critical, parental voice that says, 'You should try harder, you're not good enough.' The inner justifier has a self-righteous, childish voice that says, 'Don't blame me, it's not my fault, I did the best I could, it was the others who weren't cooperating.' One of these can drive your inner thoughts, directing how you feel about yourself. They become apparent when you reflect on your inner self-talk and begin to notice the patterns.

Kristin Neff (2011, *Self Compassion: Stop Beating Yourself Up and Leave Insecurity Behind*) explains:

> People deeply internalize their parents' criticisms, meaning that the disparaging running commentary they hear inside their own head is often a reflection of parental voices – sometimes passed down and replicated through generations. (p.25)

Sometimes you can convince yourself that the voice of the inner judge belongs to those around you. Instead of directly criticizing yourself, you imagine that all of your friends, acquaintances, family members or work colleagues are critical of you. Your feeling or thoughts will be, 'everyone thinks that I should...' or 'they think that I am...' This sort of thinking can give you much pain because you become very concerned about what other people think of you. If you can, try to work on it to remove these negative thoughts. Be kind to yourself and remind yourself regularly that everyone else is much too busy thinking about their own problems to be thinking about you.

To get rid of an inner voice that is trying to control you might seem difficult at first, but gets easier as you practise it. Sit quietly for a while, allowing your body to relax and your breathing to slow down. Remind yourself that your thoughts are not the sum total of your being. You can stand back from your thinking self. You have already stood back from your thinking self if you have noticed your inner voices. Then take yourself into a neutral position where you are in a state of impassive objectivity, and ask yourself the simple question, 'is it true?' When you stop and really look at all of the running commentary spooling through your mind, is it true what it says? Is it really true? Or is it exaggerated, misinformed, out of date or irrelevant? Make some notes in your reflective journal, to remind yourself for next time.

CHOOSING A NEUTRAL ROLE

There are many ways in which the balance of power can ebb and flow between the practitioner and patient. The practitioner has the skills, knowledge and experience of their therapy. The patient has the knowledge and experience of their body, emotions, thoughts and their symptoms. Added to these are the relationships that are brought in from the past that mask or distort the picture.

The practitioner has to find a way of detaching themselves from these relationship patterns, and assume the role of unprejudiced observer, a term used by homeopaths for the last 200 years. Returning to the Drama Triangle, there is a fourth position which is called the Leveller. This person has stepped outside of the Drama Triangle, and looks at what is going on from a neutral, unbiased and common-sense perspective. With reference to the three ego states, anyone can consciously put themselves into Adult mode, which encourages the other person to do likewise. It is much more difficult to act out the role of Child or Parent when the partner in the transaction is a calm, present, neutral Adult. When both people are in Adult mode, communication will be much more straightforward.

COMPASSION AND THE UNPREJUDICED OBSERVER

It becomes apparent that the best case-taking will be from a neutral viewpoint, without getting involved in a patient-led drama or game. This does not mean being coldly and clinically objective. For me, the three images of Leveller, Adult and unprejudiced observer all come from the same archetype of someone calm, neutral, unbiased, present and compassionate. Being unbiased means that you have no prejudgement or expectations of the patient – which allows them to just be who they are. If you are present in a mindful way, you are more likely to notice if the patient changes ego states or presents as victim; you will notice but not become involved. If you are present and compassionate, you can simply listen to them whatever they say, with an attitude of loving kindness and acceptance.

Sympathy means to feel sorry for someone. You feel no emotional involvement but rather an intellectual concern for the other's situation or suffering. Empathy echoes or mirrors the other person's suffering to a certain extent. When you feel empathy, you can get a sense of the other person's pain and link it in to the universal experiences that we have all had. Compassion takes things further; it is similar to empathy where you feel the other's pain – but it is coupled with the desire to help. Compassion reaches out to other people in a way that is proactive. The word compassion comes from the Latin, meaning 'co-suffering' or 'suffering together with'.

It is a goal to aim for, that you might not achieve with every patient, but worth working towards. If you spend time with your reflective journal, you can become a lot more aware of when you are involved in power games and when you are centred and compassionate.

Robin Youngson (2012) was a traditional doctor who worked in a paternalistic way, holding the power because he was the expert with the experience; until a patient showed him there was another way of being with those he treated. He realized the importance of being compassionate and taking time to simply be with them in a mindful way. Writing in *Time to Care: How to Love Your Patients and Your Job*, he reminds us how much we can learn from our patients:

> Before meeting Jessie, I conceived of the doctor–patient relationship as a one-way street. I was the highly trained doctor, the expert, and the person with authority and control. Caring was a one-way process. I cared for patients and I determined the process and the agenda.

> Patients didn't care for me. They were grateful, of course, they took my advice and they did what I told them. Those who didn't were 'difficult' patients or 'non-compliant'... But somehow, Jessie turned the tables on me... The relationship had become a two-way process. (p.88)

I do not want to infer that patients should be caring of practitioners. In this case, Jessie made him laugh when he was concerned about her refusal to have a blood transfusion. My interest in this story comes from Youngson's changeover from a paternalistic viewpoint where patients were judged as compliant or non-compliant, to a position in which he is learning from a patient about a cooperating relationship. We can always learn from our patients. Sometimes this learning is on a superficial level, merely fact-finding. At other times the lesson is profound, making us rethink our role as practitioners. Don't resist these lessons; reflect on them and feel appreciation for the opportunity to move forward in your own self-development.

THE KEY IS COURTESY

In learning about these relationship patterns and games, you can avoid playing them. It is more difficult for the patient to escape from them, especially if their previous experiences with other practitioners were dysfunctional. You are not in a position to teach them the models described here; it is not your job. However, when you treat your patient with courtesy and respect and you have the strong expectation that they will do likewise, you encourage a relationship that is immediately more cooperative. Then they are much more likely to give the case clearly without unconscious role-playing; and a clearer case gives you a better chance of helping them.

▌REFLECTIVE EXAMPLE

I had a new patient today: a 17-year-old pregnant girl with morning sickness, whose mother came as well to support her. There was some sort of power dynamic going on, and I'd like to unravel it. The image that comes to me is a set of Russian dolls, the foetus inside the girl, the girl inside/protected by the mother – and I was on the outside.

The mother was very protective towards the daughter, and sometimes actually stopped me asking questions, because she said they would upset the daughter. At other times she answered for the daughter. It's true, the daughter cried very easily, tears rolling down her cheeks in a sort of helpless way – and it was lovely to see how much the mother cared for her. The boyfriend had abandoned her, and her mother had taken over. In terms of the Drama Triangle, she has rescued her daughter in a big way. The mother is the Rescuer, the daughter is the Victim and the boyfriend is/was the Persecutor.

The problem is, the pregnant daughter is my patient and yet I seem to be writing as much about the mother. The image that comes to me now is that the mother is standing between me and my patient like a mother tiger. Does she see me as another Persecutor?

I think I should have asked to see the daughter on her own, but they were such a tight unit that I let the mother stay. Interesting, but it was a mistake. Who does the mother remind me of? The image that comes to me now is that of a schoolteacher; the old-fashioned, very strict type of schoolteacher. In terms of the three ego states, she is definitely a critical Parent towards me, and probably a nurturing Parent towards her daughter. The daughter is very much in Child mode, probably free Child; she is spontaneous considering the unplanned pregnancy and the tears.

Where does that leave me? Was I in Adult mode? It doesn't sound like it if I see the mother as a tiger or a strict schoolteacher. Most likely I was in compensated Child, obedient to the mother's strict Parent. No wonder I was on the outside of the three Russian dolls!

What I did well

I asked as many questions as I could and felt I had enough information to make a reasonable prescription. I arranged for another appointment in two weeks, with a phone call in between.

What I didn't do so well

I got held at bay by the protective mother (another image: hunting dogs). I didn't set up a good working relationship with the daughter. I said all the right things, but I think I didn't get enough eye contact with her to really form a relationship. The mother kept diverting my attention to herself.

Action plan

Try to separate them next time! Or tell the mother that I got a lot of valuable information from her last time, and this time I'd like to just hear from my patient.

EXERCISE: NOTICING YOUR INNER VOICES

Imagine that you and a friend or relative have had a long car drive, and now you're tired and wishing for a hot shower and comfortable bed. An argument breaks out between the two of you about where to stay or whether to eat first. It becomes quite heated, and then fades away because both of you are tired. Working with your reflective journal, write down what the voices in your head would be saying while you continue that drive. Would you find yourself furiously criticizing the other person and justifying your own position (your inner justifier)? Or would you be angry with yourself for taking part in the row (your inner judge)?

Then imagine that you have been asked to do a presentation in front of 24 people at work, and you make a mess of it. Write down what the different voices in your head would be saying this time. Would the inner judge or the inner justifier have the loudest voice? What do they say? Which voice is most familiar for you?

EXERCISE: YOUR FREE CHILD AND YOUR NURTURING PARENT

Think back to the last time you expressed your free Child. Looking through old photos can be helpful, because as a free Child you would have been having fun, expressing yourself spontaneously or even doing something unconventional. You might have been with a group of friends, going to a party, watching a game or simply on holiday. Free time often encourages the free Child to emerge. Then think back to the last time you expressed your nurturing Parent, choosing a time when you were not actually parenting your children or grandchildren. If you have chosen to be part of the caring professions as a practitioner, you probably took the role of the nurturing Parent very recently.

How does it feel being in these two roles? Are you familiar with them or are you more comfortable as compromised Child or the critical Parent?

EXERCISE: SELF-COMPASSION

Think back to any family discussion or heated argument between friends that you were part of. The Drama Triangle was probably present, either mildly or played out with full theatrical energy. Which part did you take? Did you remain with the same part or did you shift into another role? Was this a typical role for you or were you surprised?

Working with this example and with another one if you wish, see if you can identify which is your favoured role in the Drama Triangle. How do you feel about what you have discovered? None of the three roles is particularly flattering and you might not like what you have discovered. Can you trace back to what your family life was like for you under the age of eight or nine? What dynamics were present, that might have pushed you into one particular role? For example, children that become carers at an early age for disabled parents can become Rescuers as adults.

Now write some soothing words to yourself in your reflective journal. Remind yourself that it is okay to be a player in the Drama Triangle and over time you will get better and better at noticing when you are involved. Forgive yourself for the number of times you were responding within the Drama Triangle in the past without realizing it. Create an image of yourself as a teenager, bouncing around the three roles just for the drama of it, and gently laugh at and forgive yourself. It's okay, many people are like that as teenagers. Don't put yourself under any pressure to change, but gently tell yourself that soon you will get the hang of being a Leveller. You can't say when exactly, but you can be certain that once you have opened your awareness it won't take long.

Chapter 4

SAFETY AND THE WORKING AGREEMENT

Many alternative practitioners are self-employed, and put a lot of effort into building up their practice. But a sizeable number of patients don't return after the first or second appointment. Why is that? Have they been cured? Among the homeopathic community the assumption is usually that the first prescription was not effective, and that the patient is trying another route. Homeopaths compensate by studying new books and new methodologies, in order to make better prescriptions. Practitioners in other therapies feel equally depressed with non-returners, because they have worked hard to help the patient.

On the other extreme, I'm sure we've all experienced patients who come back with great regularity, despite what appears to be no change in symptoms after several treatments. Are these patients simply hypochondriacs? Or is their loyalty misplaced because they see us as a friend or supportive parent?

My theory is that patient return rates are influenced by how comfortable and secure they feel as a patient under your care, regardless of results. I suggest that patients make rapid decisions about whether they feel comfortable with you and can trust you. People read body language far faster than they listen to words, and a short time in your company lets them know whether they feel safe.

It can be helpful to look at Maslow's (1943) hierarchy of needs (see Box 4.1) to understand the patient's needs for the duration of the consultation. Maslow proposed that human beings are motivated by certain basic needs, and as each need is satisfied they will move onto the next one, working towards self-actualization. There are five levels of needs which he originally showed in a pyramid diagram with the more basic needs at the bottom. It is a simplistic model and was not well-researched (Maslow researched only 18 people that he considered to be self-actualized). However, it gives us a useful framework.

BOX 4.1 MASLOW'S HIERARCHY OF NEEDS

- Needs for self-actualization
- Needs for self-esteem and esteem from others
- Needs for love, affection and belonging
- Safety needs
- Physiological needs

MASLOW'S FIRST LEVEL: PHYSIOLOGICAL NEEDS

The most basic needs are the primitive, biological needs of oxygen, food, water and a relatively consistent body temperature. A patient who has travelled some distance might be in need of a toilet or a glass of water when they arrive. Some patients are particularly sensitive to heat, cold or drafts and cannot feel comfortable until the climate has been readjusted. Young children who are brought to a consultation immediately after school will often need a drink and snack before they are willing to cooperate. As the practitioner, you usually attend to these physiological needs without thinking, offering water, directing to the bathroom, and checking if the patient is comfortable in their seat or with the temperature of the room. It is the parent's responsibility to provide sustenance for their children, but you might need to remind them.

Most people need a short breathing space between their arrival and the start of the consultation, especially if it is the first appointment. It is as if their body has entered the clinic, but their mind has not arrived yet. The mind is still taken up with details of the journey, and making a rapid assessment of both you and your clinic. The patient needs a couple of minutes to arrive fully and become grounded in the consultation room before they are ready to give information about their condition.

You probably respond to this automatically by asking about the patient's journey, or talking about the weather in order to provide breathing space for the patient.

MASLOW'S SECOND LEVEL: SAFETY NEEDS

The second of Maslow's hierarchy of needs is safety. Without a sense of safety, the patient will be uncomfortable and might be unable to give the case satisfactorily, leading to a misdiagnosis. If they feel unsafe, their sense of vulnerability will increase and their power to understand and remember your instructions will decrease.

Lack of safety might be triggered by unfulfilled physiological needs, such as the patient that is too shy to ask for fresh air, but feels uncomfortable in the stuffy room. It could be triggered by the environment, such as realizing the receptionist can hear everything, because you can both hear everything she says. Your non-verbal communication can make a patient feel uneasy, such as the practitioner who invades their personal space before they are ready – even if they have come for a massage. If the patient misunderstands the treatment protocol they might feel very uncomfortable, such as not realizing they would have to undress down to underwear for the treatment. A feeling of lack of safety might be a long-term, chronic condition arising from the patient's own experience or delusions.

Take a few minutes to think back over your own experiences as a patient going to see a new doctor, dentist, hospital or alternative practitioner. Have you had the experience of not understanding the 'ground rules' of the clinic and feeling rather uneasy, foolish or vulnerable? You might have assumed that the routines would be exactly the same as your previous practitioner's, and it took you a few minutes to readjust to the new rules. For example, do you know which of the alternative practices need the shoes to be taken off and which of them leave the shoes on?

As a practitioner you can increase the feeling of safety for the patient through your courtesy and respect as they arrive, such as reassuring the patient on first meeting them that they have arrived at the correct address and they are expected, or introducing yourself. You can take the patient's coat and hang it up, show them where they should sit or find out if they have any physiological needs. You can begin with the familiar, routine questions such as the patient's address, contact numbers, e-mail address and date of birth.

You can further reassure the patient and encourage their trust through your non-verbal communication. You can deliberately make use of non-aggressive eye contact, quiet smiles, soft, gentle movements, open body posture and encouraging nods. Sometimes we instinctively change our non-verbal communication. With certain patients I have found myself changing my voice into the gentle, deep and slow reassuring tone that I would use with a sick child or frightened animal. There is certainly no disrespect intended and it happens intuitively, before I have time to think about it.

Writing in *The Inner Consultation: How to Develop an Effective and Intuitive Consulting Style*, Roger Neighbour (2005) suggests that practitioners should deliberately match the patient's non-verbal communication style. He points out that people who are close do this to create a rapport:

> They are talking about the same topic in similar terms, understanding each other's nuances and idiosyncrasies, using awareness of each other's eye contact and speech inflection to synchronize their conversation. Their voices will be similarly paced and pitched, matched for volume, rhythm and modulation. In their facial expressions, the hand movements, the alignment of their torsos and the disposition of their limbs they closely resemble each other. (p.137)

Once the patient has settled, if this is the first appointment you should briefly explain your main expectations of your practitioner–patient relationship. This is called contracting or making a working agreement.

Working agreements or contracts are familiar to everyone. These are the agreements (often in writing) between two people or a group of people about what sort of relationship they intend to have together. Marriage is formalized by a contract. When joining a business, you start with a contract that you sign stating the hours that you will work and the amount you will be paid. In many schools in Britain there is a three-part contract between the student, the teacher and the parents to agree on expectations, responsibilities, behaviour and cooperation. If a builder is going to do some work for you, he will send a notification with the details of the work to be done and the estimated fee.

BOX 4.2 THE WORKING AGREEMENT BETWEEN PRACTITIONER AND PATIENT...

- clarifies the patient's expectations
- informs the patient about the nature of the treatment
- creates a common goal with clear time limits and fees
- allocates responsibilities
- reassures about confidentiality
- defines the boundaries of the relationship.

Having a working agreement clarifies expectations on both sides. It is an opportunity for you to explain what you can provide and the patient to see if this is what they want. It allows both of you to create a common goal that you will work towards and it sets out who takes responsibility for what. It should also clarify where boundaries lie, although frequently this is the weakest part of the contract and more attention should be given to it (see Chapter 9 on boundaries).

Working agreements can be fixed or flexible. A fixed working agreement allows no negotiation. It is a clear statement of what you can provide and what is expected from the patient. It is usually available on the website or as a flyer for the patient to read before they arrive. It might begin with a simple description of what treatments or therapies you can provide, followed by details about what the patient can expect, such as, the length of time for an average consultation, the fees, the cancellation policy, your working hours, who to contact outside of your working hours, and confidentiality.

A fixed working agreement is usually done in writing so that the patient can take home a copy, and in some countries they are asked to sign a copy to go on file. A flexible working agreement is one that has been negotiated between you and your individual patient; a record is kept in the patient folder or given to the patient.

Most working agreements have a fixed element, such as fees and working hours, but are still flexible enough to create a common goal that is negotiated between you and your patient. For example, a patient comes to an osteopath for the first time, because they have stiff muscles in the back and shoulder after doing home improvements.

They have been told by their friends that one treatment will work miracles. The osteopath has discovered through experience that this sort of injury usually takes two or three appointments, and he recommends using acupuncture on a couple of points as well. He wants the patient to do a few specific, regular exercises between appointments. These very different expectations need to be spoken about and negotiated, in order to create a common goal. It will only take a few minutes, and the rest of the working agreement can be given to the patient as a handout or flyer.

The key to a successful working relationship is sharing the responsibility between you and your patient. This starts with the case taking. You provide your knowledge and skills whilst the patient needs to give adequate information about their condition to enable you to do your work. The patient shows commitment by taking any prescriptions as instructed and following your recommendations for exercise, sleep or nutrition between appointments. If they feel it is unlikely they will be able to do this you can negotiate what is more practical for them. Finally, you need to advise the patient not to lose contact with their regular doctor or hospital, and any medication should not be changed or terminated without medical advice.

Confidentiality is often taken as a given because it is written into every code of ethics, but it's reassuring if you put it into the working agreement as well. You will need to remind the patient of confidentiality if you're taking the case into supervision; you can reassure them that there will be no identifying details given to the supervisor such as their name or occupation. This might happen because you need extra help with the case, or when a student practitioner is working with a supervisor for their graduation cases.

When running groups or workshops, I find that if we spend time on the first two steps of Maslow's hierarchy the group will run together smoothly and confidently. Again, the physiological issues need to be dealt with first. People need to know where to find the toilets and when their lunch break will be. Then we move on to the working agreement, and I always get the group to negotiate their own working agreement. I have very strong expectations that they can do this together, so I facilitate rather than lead. However, I do check that they have included empathy, respect and confidentiality. We leave the written working agreement in full view all day on a whiteboard or flipchart.

THE SESSION CONTRACT

The session contract is a little reminder in which the practitioner signposts what is going to happen during the consultation. For the patient, coming to a new practitioner for the first time, it is not always obvious what will happen during the first appointment. Much as we would like the patient to have done some background reading, they often have no idea what to expect and have just come because of a recommendation. You will have to explain what will happen (see Figure 4.1).

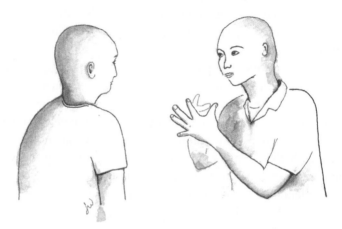

FIGURE 4.1: EXPLAIN OR NEGOTIATE THE WORKING AGREEMENT

Some alternative therapies involve hands-on treatment, such as massage, shiatsu or Reiki; some involve instruments such as the needles of an acupuncturist; and some result in a prescription, such as herbalism, Chinese medicine or homeopathy. If you can take a few minutes to explain (signpost) what will happen during the consultation, you will increase the patient's sense of security and they will be more compliant. It need not be wordy or take long and can be as simple as telling them how long the treatment will last today or what sort of questions will be asked during the consultation.

For example, an acupuncturist might explain to the patient that they will start with the medical history working from a questionnaire. After this they will ask the patient to undress down to their underwear, and lie face up on the treatment couch.

As a homeopath I have always taken care to explain to patients the holistic nature of homeopathy. The first appointment usually takes one and a half hours, during which I ask questions about the presenting symptoms, general physical characteristics such as food desires or sleep patterns, and their thoughts and feelings. Before we begin I explain to the patient that although this information doesn't seem relevant to their particular symptoms, it helps me to choose the best remedy for them. Prescriptions are chosen to match the individual person and their personality, in comparison with conventional medicine where prescriptions are chosen to match the symptoms of the illness or disease. The 200-year-old method of homeopathic consultation gets the patient talking in depth about themselves, in a way that is probably only mirrored in counselling or psychotherapy.

MAKING A WORKING AGREEMENT WITH CHILDREN

Making a working agreement when the patient is a child is usually done with the parent or carer, but a separate, simplified agreement can be made with the child. Some children are nervous as they have been told they are going to see the doctor or hospital, when they are being brought to an alternative practitioner. They need reassurance with a light touch.

I suggest that you negotiate an agreement with the parent first, and then take a few minutes to introduce yourself directly to the child; with eye contact if they are not too shy. Explain that they have been brought to see you so that you can help with their symptoms and this might mean a lot of questions for the grown-up. Tell the child that they can answer some questions if they want, or they can play with the toys on the floor. If the child shows interest, you can begin with asking them how old they are.

RE-CONTRACTING

If a patient finds it difficult to keep to the working agreement, they can be gently reminded of it, such as the patient who misses an appointment and might need the cancellation policy to be mentioned again.

The working agreement can be changed or re-contracted at any time by either person or both. Some practitioners like to make an initial arrangement of three or four appointments, followed by a review. At the review, both of you can contribute your observations and thoughts about how well the patient is progressing towards their goal. Then according to how this is going, a new arrangement is set up.

In my monthly supervision groups for practitioners there are regular issues about patients pushing the boundaries such as: 'They forgot to bring enough cash again!', 'They asked me to treat both children in the same session!', 'They expected me to prescribe over the phone without seeing the patient!', 'They asked for a home visit when I know they're perfectly capable of coming to my clinic!' With all of these, I ask what was in the original working agreement to see if we can identify whether the patient is truly at fault or whether something has happened to make the practitioner relax their boundaries (see Chapter 9 for more on boundaries). Then we can start to consider how the patient can be reminded of the working agreement – or if this was lacking, how to introduce a contract.

A student that I was supervising found his patient so much better at the second appointment that he told her she didn't need to come back for another six weeks or longer. On checking whether this was okay with the patient, he realized too late that she was feeling abandoned by him. While discussing this in supervision, I agreed with him that there was no point in seeing the patient while all was well, but he must make it very clear that he still supported her. I suggested that he write to her, congratulating her on all her improvements and explaining that was why he didn't need to see her. He should tell her that she could come back at any time sooner than six weeks if she needed to. This would clarify the re-contract for the patient and give her room to negotiate if she needed to.

MASLOW'S THIRD LEVEL: NEEDS OF LOVE, AFFECTION AND BELONGINGNESS

When the patient has been satisfied in their needs for physiological comfort and safety, they are ready to open up in the consultation. At this level their dominant needs are around love, affection and belongingness. This is the third level, at the centre of Maslow's hierarchy of needs.

Once they have understood the working agreement and have been told what to expect from the consultation and the first treatment, the patient starts to relax and can give the case clearly and honestly.

If your body language and interview skills continue to show respect, understanding and compassion, the patient will reveal more and more which in turn enables you to work to a higher level. Then the treatment goes well, and the prescription is well chosen.

In terms of the practitioner–patient relationship the word 'love' is normally avoided in case it encourages an inappropriate relationship with the patient. The love felt in the consultation has nothing to do with sexuality, friendship or even the love of a parent for their child. The love felt by the practitioner for the patient is low-key and has a cerebral and spiritual nature and might be described as affection, loving-kindness or unconditional positive regard. This love has elements of intimacy, respect and compassion. It recognizes the universal aspects of the human condition in the individual and does not judge or compare. It simply accepts that the patient did the best they could at the time. It is expressed through your attentive listening, your body language that shows interest and invites the patient to say more, and your facial expressions that show compassion and your genuine wish to understand them.

In my own experience with new patients or new supervisees, I feel a gentle interest or curiosity as they arrive, and I feel calm or slightly controlling as we work our way through the two initial stages of Maslow's hierarchy, those of physiological needs and safety needs. Then when I start to take the case, after five or ten minutes I look up from my note-taking, refocus on the patient and see that they look completely beautiful. That is the moment when I know my compassion and loving kindness have kicked in, and that I am walking beside the patient rather than simply observing them.

On the patient's side, they have been made to feel secure and safe through the attention to their physiological and safety needs, and are starting to feel a sense of ownership of the treatment plan. Trust is being built up and regard is felt on both sides. The patient feels a sense of belonging and being held, contained or even loved, which nourishes them. This can happen as early as ten or fifteen minutes into the session and I suggest it is one of the deciding factors about whether the patient returns for future treatments.

MASLOW'S FOURTH LEVEL: ESTEEM

Maslow's fourth level is about self-esteem, confidence, self-respect and respect by others. In terms of the consultation, this is the case-taking stage where information is gathered. I suggest this is the deepest acknowledgement of the patient by you. We could say, it is the acknowledgement of the patient's inner, perfect soul self or inner spirit body. The patient feels valued by you, and their sense of self-worth increases. They begin to feel they deserve well-being. It is like a blessing or the sunshine warming them. The patient turns towards the sunshine, opens up and is ready for healing.

The fourth level often blends easily into Maslow's fifth level: that of self-actualization, which is where healing happens. Self-actualization is a fulfilling of potential, enabling the patient to become more of a whole person, and can be achieved through alternative therapies that offer holistic treatment.

CREATING THE RIGHT CONDITIONS FOR HEALING

I have linked Maslow's hierarchy of needs to the building of the relationship between practitioner and patient. Writing a whole chapter on this makes it sound like there is a lot to be done, but in practice it takes five to ten minutes of the first consultation, with brief reminders at other times. It doesn't always happen in the same order as Maslow, and if any stage has been missed, it can be returned to at another time. The importance is to create the right conditions for healing, where the patient feels safe enough, respected enough and understood enough.

REFLECTIVE EXAMPLE

What happened?

My new patient this morning was incredibly talkative. She started telling me all of her symptoms as soon as she walked through the door and continued talking while she took off her coat and sat down. She had symptoms, she had her opinions about her symptoms, she had doctors and hospital reports and her opinions about them; she had a lot to say. I tried to interrupt at the beginning in order to do my working agreement, but she just kept going, hardly even drawing a breath.

So what?

I decided to wait until she had run out of steam, but hardly had I started speaking when she interrupted me with, 'Oh, and another thing, I must tell you before I forget...' I tried to take notes but couldn't keep pace with what she was saying.

She had no idea of time and started to overrun the appointment. I gathered my courage and interrupted her, saying that we would have to end. I read back to her what I considered to be the main elements of the case, which was a mistake because it started her off again, and then I had to ask her to leave because my next patient was waiting.

So what?

I completely failed to take her through the working agreement. She might, or might not have read my terms and conditions on the website. I wasn't able to tell her what my prognosis and instructions were for the following month. I didn't even make the next appointment. I have never been so overwhelmed by a patient's loquacity.

So what?

I felt overwhelmed, I felt unprofessional, I felt I didn't have any solid ground to stand on, I felt helpless in the face of this tidal wave, I had doubts whether I could work with her without her pushing all of my boundaries. I'm a bit irritated with myself for asking her whether I had understood her well enough. It just invited more words.

What if?

What if I had made more of an effort to control the session? Looking back on it, I don't think she would have minded. I'm sure other people have to interrupt her or be her timekeeper.

What if she is like this for every appointment? What if she starts phoning me between appointments? I would have a hard job keeping her contained.

What if?

What if I had powerfully interrupted her in the first five minutes, and insisted on us doing a working agreement? Again, I don't think she would have minded. It's not my style to dominate the consultation or interrupt patients, but I suppose there will always be exceptions to the rule.

So what?

I could phone her and say, 'There are a few things I need to check with you before we proceed.' But she would probably have a dozen fresh symptoms that she's just remembered that she wants to tell me. I would need to have the strength to say to her, 'Tell me any other symptoms next time you see me, but at the moment I need to discuss how we're going to work together.'

So what?

I could e-mail her my terms and conditions. She may not read them, but to avoid this I could ask her, 'Please read through this and e-mail me your agreement before our next appointment.' That would be a strong statement of my boundaries. I could keep a copy of these e-mails in the file.

So what?

Playing devil's advocate, I could e-mail her to offer my apologies saying, 'On consideration I don't think I'm able to help you, so rather than to waste your time or money, we won't be making another appointment.' I don't have to treat every patient that comes. I can say no, because I am self-employed. But having written that, I realize that I do want to work with her and it will be an interesting learning experience.

I think I will e-mail her my terms and conditions.

EXERCISE: MAKING A WORKING AGREEMENT

Think ahead to your next holiday with family or friends, or the next time you go to visit someone. Make a working agreement with them. (I have always found this an excellent plan when going on holiday with teenagers.) You might want to include:

- time issues, such as when you will arrive, when you're going to have meals and what time everyone plans to get up in the morning

- responsibilities, such as who will cook, who will choose the restaurant, who will carry the bags and who will bring mosquito cream

- individual desires and needs versus group activities, such as how to decide what everyone does each day, and how to arrange free time

- communication with others in the group, such as informing others where you're going and when you will return

- money issues, such as how you will pay for group activities and who will pay for snacks and souvenirs.

EXERCISE: YOU CAN ALWAYS RE-CONTRACT

Supposing a patient came to you on a regular basis over a couple of years. She was pleased with your work, and being a sociable, chatty sort of person, she started handing out your cards and referring you to all of her acquaintances. You really appreciate her enthusiasm and the new clients that she is sending your way. However, over time you gradually realize that she is asking for a lot of special favours in return, such as a last-minute, 'quick' appointment in your lunch break, or that she will pay you the next time she sees you. It dawns on you that she is eliciting these favours in return for the new patients that she has sent you. You have been advised to re-contract with her before her demands increase. When would you speak to her? (the next time she asks for a favour or cold call her?) and what would you say to her?

EXERCISE: MAKING YOURSELF FEEL SAFE

How do you make yourself feel safe? Do you have any techniques that you use for difficult situations such as going to the dentist, your first day at college, speaking in public or walking into a room full of strangers at a party.

Self-compassion can shift your thinking and your emotions from anxiety to acceptance. Tell yourself that it's okay, you're doing really well. Remember that you are not the only one to feel like this, it's normal and most people have felt like this at some time or other. Remind yourself that you have survived on previous occasions, and frequently it's not as bad as you might anticipate.

Mindfulness is the term for holding your thoughts and feelings in the present moment, without anticipating the future or bemoaning the past. Take five or ten minutes to sit quietly, with your eyes resting or closed and quietly listen to your breathing. Don't try to change anything, just notice your breathing and accept the rhythm of it, whether fast or slow, deep or shallow. Then gently, slowly, silently explore your body without moving, just noticing any symptoms of anxiety and accepting them from your position of unprejudiced observer. Notice any physical symptoms such as increased warmth or cold, rumblings in your stomach or the dryness or increased saliva in your mouth. Don't judge yourself in any way for having these sensations, just notice them and allow them. They are what they are and that's okay.

Chapter 5

MINDFULNESS

Mindfulness refers to bringing your attentive awareness to the present moment's experience and accepting whatever there is without judgement. This is the opposite of concentration which is forcing your thinking mind to remain with one issue over time. Concentration includes investigation, study, analysis and evaluation. In contrast, mindfulness asks you to quieten the mind and open the heart in a way that is non-judgemental, accepting, compassionate and present to what is happening right now. It is a learned ability to sit in the present experience, without reference to the past or future.

BEING IN THE PRESENT

How often do you really look at the view out of your window, and how often do you gaze across it absentmindedly while considering inner pictures created out of memories and imagination? It is an interesting experiment to take the time to really be in the present, noticing and enjoying the view out of the window – holding your mind in simple appreciation like a child, without judging or analysing what you see. As soon as you start to think about it, you will probably stop looking at it and re-enter your own internal world. Mindfulness will never completely stop the mind roaming and ruminating; but it is the practice of gently bringing your attention back to the here and now; in this case back to the view out of the window again.

As an experiment, try spending the next five minutes mindfully cleaning your computer. Take a soft cloth or a tissue and slowly wipe over the machine, noticing the different colours and textures but without analysing. Your hands know what to do, so you don't need to concentrate or follow instructions. Just watch your hands as they do this basic task, and keep yourself in the present moment, where it is peaceful. When your mind wanders (which it will) just gently bring it back to the awareness of the present moment again.

I was asked to do a mindful meditation session with a group of students. I gave everyone two raisins to hold, and asked them to sit quietly and observe their own breathing pattern without judgement or desire to change it. As most of them were sitting with their eyes closed, I asked them to delicately touch the two raisins with their fingertips and do a gentle examination of the wrinkly surface. I asked them to quietly and appreciatively notice their sense of touch. I waited in silence while they did this. Then I asked them to smell the raisins by holding them up to the nose and inhaling deeply. Next I asked them to open their eyes and really look at the raisins, absorbing their shape, colour and texture. Then I suggested they put the raisins in their mouth and gently roll them around without chewing while they noticed the flavour, sweetness and texture. Finally I asked them to eat the raisins and notice the noise that came from chewing and swallowing.

Working through the senses encouraged them to carefully observe the fullness of what it meant to eat a raisin, being open to the experience and being present in the moment.

Some of the students doing this mindful meditation for the first time found it quite difficult to keep the mind quiet, because they were anxious about 'doing it right'. But there are no rules to mindful meditation; there is simply the guideline that you should notice, be aware and accept. Some of the students were in a deep meditative state until I asked them to open their eyes and look at the raisins. After that their attention wandered. When doing mindfulness practice this doesn't need to be interpreted or analysed. It is just something to notice and be aware of. It would be the same if some pain or sensation in the body takes you away from the present. Just notice it and gently come back again to your 'anchor', whether this is being aware of your breathing, looking at the view out of the window or eating a raisin. Gently come back to the present as many times as it takes.

You will have experienced being fully in the present moment numerous times and although each experience was probably quite brief, you will remember several of them because they filled you with a sense of peaceful, expanded exhilaration. These are the times where you are completely in the flow of the moment, without thought or judgement, just being and experiencing, like seeing a magnificent sunset, dancing to your favourite piece of music, listening to a wonderful song, watching your team scoring the winning goal, playing a sport when you and your team-mates are perfectly coordinated, running into the sea on the first day of your holiday or holding a newborn baby in your arms.

With mindfulness practice, you learn to have more and more of these moments when you are just in the experience of the current moment, without thinking about it and without comparing it to the past or imagining the future. Paul Gilbert (2009) writes in *The Compassionate Mind*, 'Mindfulness brings us fully alive to the *now* of our conscious existence, the only place we actually exist!' (p.250, italics in the original).

Being totally present and slowing down your thoughts can allow you to observe yourself with calm detachment. Neff (2011) writes, 'Mindfulness is sometimes seen as a form of "meta-awareness," which means awareness of awareness' (p.86). She compares it to watching a movie, an experience where sometimes you can become so engrossed that you are living the plot alongside the actors – and at other times, you are aware of yourself as one of the people watching the film. She goes on to say:

> When you focus on the fact that you are having certain thoughts and feelings, you are no longer lost in their storyline. You can wake up and look around you, taking an outsider's perspective on your experience. (p.87)

This outsider's perspective or meta-awareness is a major element of mindfulness. If you are absorbed by the feelings and sensations of what is happening, it is as if you are too close to the fire. The noise and the heat of it will trigger your fight–flight response and you will become impatient, irritable, frightened or angry – and highly stressed. If you move away to a cooler place you can get a wider angle viewpoint and can put the fire into context with the rest of the landscape. The further back you go, the larger the panorama you can see and the fire becomes an insignificant spot on the horizon.

MINDFULNESS AND SCIENCE

Mindfulness comes from Eastern philosophies such as Buddhism, Taoism and yoga and it has been around in the West for about 40 years. Mindfulness-Based Stress Reduction (MBSR) was introduced by Jon Kabat-Zinn in 1979 after he did a survey of doctor's cure rates with patients (Santorelli 1999). The doctors estimated it could be as low as 20 per cent and Kabat-Zinn proposed that he run groups for those patients who were not cured, teaching them the practice of mindfulness, yoga and other self-help techniques. These groups are now being run all over the USA and around the world and thousands of people have completed the eight-week course. MBSR training has been found to reduce stress, reduce pain, raise self-awareness, enhance emotional intelligence and generally improve the quality of life.

In the last decade, mindfulness has been scientifically examined and proven. One example of this is the Mindful Attention Awareness Scale (MAAS) (Brown and Ryan 2003). This comes in the form of a self-assessment questionnaire that has 15 statements about your awareness during the day. For example, 'I could be experiencing some emotion and not be conscious of it until sometime later' or 'I rush through activities without being really attentive to them.' You are given six choices of reply to these statements: almost always, very frequently, somewhat frequently, somewhat infrequently, very infrequently and almost never. From these your mindfulness can be assessed.

For you the benefits are numerous: you will become a lot calmer and less stressed, which means you're less likely to have burnout. You will enjoy your work more and do far less mental juggling. You will become more open, adaptable and easy going. You might become more intuitive and let go of the need to rationalize everything. As a practitioner you will approach each patient with an open minded, loving curiosity. You will let go of expectations and prejudice and simply enjoy each patient for what they are. Your listening skills will improve and you will be more present for the patient. Youngson (2012) observes:

> As my connection with patients has deepened, I experience precious moments of stillness, heightened awareness, compassion, and loving-kindness. These practices are meditations in themselves. (p.67)

From the patient's perspective, they will feel really listened to, which in turn helps them to open up and tell you really useful information about themselves. The consultation becomes more effective as the patient uncovers their core issues; and you will be able to work on a deeper level. The patients will develop trust and return regularly for follow-up appointments.

Santorelli (1999) writes:

My own experience suggests that the willingness to stop and be present leads to seeing and relating to circumstances and events with more clarity and directness. Out of this directness seems to emerge deeper understanding or insight into the life unfolding within and before us. Such insights allows us the possibility of choosing responses most called for by the situation rather than those reactively driven by fear, habit, or long-standing training. (p.32)

The same is observed by Douglas Falkner (2013), in his article 'Back to the source, the power of objective observation':

In the process of developing our skills in objective observation, we must also learn to engage our capacity to be present, drawing our awareness into alignment with ourselves and with the living being before us. This alignment produces a kind of resonance in the consultation room between homeopath and patient. This resonant connection is crucial if we want to delve deeply and underlies the alchemy of healing and transformation. It can be said that in achieving this kind of inner resonance and presence, we and our patients become engaged in the present moment with the process of investigation. It is this very process that will eventually lead to healing and transformation. (p.15)

PRACTISING MINDFULNESS

There are many different ways of learning mindfulness, but they all depend upon regular practice. Like any other skill, mindfulness can be understood in theory but needs to be practised until it is fully embraced as a way of being. The success of the MBSR courses is due to both the experiential element in class where the whole group practises and shares their experiences *and* the daily practice at home. With regards to choosing how you want to learn mindfulness, you could choose several methods and create your own mindfulness learning program. You might like a long, slow meditation three or four times a week, together with mindful walking for ten or fifteen minutes as part of your journey to work. Or you might choose to do the body scan first thing in the morning while lying in bed, followed by mindful cleaning of teeth, showering or shaving, followed by a mindful meal every day. There are any number of combinations.

THE BODY SCAN

One way to practise mindfulness is through doing a body scan. For this, you should lie down on a bed or on the floor with cushions or sit up if you prefer. Settle yourself into your position and take a few relaxing breaths. Starting with your left foot, bring your attention to your toes and simply notice any sensations, such as heat, cold, tickling, pain, or the touch of fabric. The sensations might be inside or outside of the toes. You don't need to analyse, and you don't need to do anything about the sensations you notice; just acknowledge them. Progress from your toes to the ball of your foot, your heel, your calves and your knees, slowly acknowledging all the sensations until you reach the top of your leg.

When you have fully acknowledged your left leg, breathe right down into the toes for a few breaths. Then start with the right leg following the same pattern. When both legs have been fully acknowledged, work your way up the back of the body and then the front. Each time you will breathe fully into the part that you have been observing before moving to the next part of the body. The arms can be done separately or together, then the neck, scalp and face. Finally, imagine your whole body as your lungs, breathing in through the top of your head and out through your feet; then entering through your feet and going out through the top of your head.

MEDITATION

Mindfulness can be developed through a regular practice of meditation, for ten to fifteen minutes every day. There are different ways of doing meditation and this example is taken from the Buddhist tradition. You might choose a different method. Begin by sitting on an upright chair with your feet on the floor or sit cross-legged on the floor. Your eyes should be open but unfocused and looking downward. Your hands should be placed palm down on your legs. You begin by gently concentrating on the breath and noticing your pattern of breathing without attempting to change anything. This becomes a sort of anchor that you can return to again and again each time your mind wanders.

As you practise this meditation, you might start to notice how often your mind wanders, and how you can gently remove each thought as it comes – or simply wait until the thought has passed.

Don't chastise yourself for thinking; it's going to happen anyway. The aim is not to stop thinking completely but to notice what is going on in your body and mind. In noticing, you become an unprejudiced observer of yourself. Gradually you will learn to relax the mind by allowing gaps of silence between each thought, just by returning to attend to the breath.

Gilbert (2009) emphasizes noticing the thinking and then returning to focusing on the breath:

> So we need to train the mind, and the only thing that is important in this training is *not to try to create anything*. You are *not* trying to create a state of relaxation. You are *not* trying to force your mind to clear itself of thoughts – which is impossible anyway. All you're doing is *allowing* yourself to playfully and gently notice when your mind wanders and then, with kindness and gentleness, bring your attention back into focus on your breathing. That's it: *notice* and *return*. (p.256, italics in original)

MINDFULNESS IN NATURE

Mindfulness can be linked to a walk that you take regularly, but please take care when crossing roads. To walk mindfully, you can allow your stride to slow down and increase your awareness of all of your senses. Notice the sounds around you of other people, birdsong, machinery, animals or vehicles. Don't think about them or try to analyse them, just observe them. Be aware of the colours, shapes and patterns of the trees, plants, wildlife, other people or buildings and enjoy them for what they are. Notice the odours and perfumes, without labelling them as pleasant or unpleasant, such as roses, freshly cut grass or an overflowing rubbish bin. Try touching some things, such as overhanging leaves from a tree, coarse brickwork or the texture of bark. If thoughts come, let them pass away and come back into the present again.

Be aware of the weather and general temperature around you. Is there sunshine, wind, mist, clouds, rain or snow? Notice what impact these have on you and your physical comfort (see Figure 5.1).

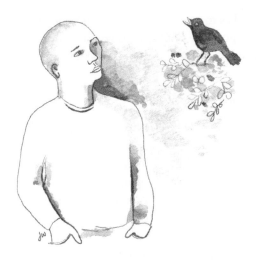

FIGURE 5.1: TAKE TIME OUT TO ENJOY THE MOMENT

LISTENING AWARENESS

If you are stuck in a queue, you can relax your visual focus and activate your listening awareness, noticing sounds such as footsteps, vehicles, shopping carts, music or people talking; but do not concentrate on any particular person's conversation. Just be fully aware of the ebb and flow of sounds around you, without trying to think about them. This mindfulness exercise I have found particularly effective in airports, where people can speak in any language from around the world. For me the international chatter is just some interesting sounds that I can listen to but do not need to interpret. I have found that with mindfulness, standing in a queue becomes relaxing rather than frustrating.

DOING ROUTINE ACTIONS MINDFULLY

Try to link mindfulness with some of your routine activities, for example every time you go through a door, clean your teeth or every time you wash the dishes. Slow down the action, and do it purposely, completely aware of all of the senses. Slow motion in movies is often used as a metaphor for heightened senses. For example, you can be mindful every time you go through a door. As you approach it, notice the colour, shape, size and texture of it, feel the shape and temperature of the door handle, observe the amount of pressure or strength it takes to release the catch, smell the little rush of air as you just begin to push the door, and as you fully open the door, look with frank curiosity at what is at the other side.

OBSERVE LIKE AN ALIEN

I have borrowed this exercise from Gilbert (2009). Imagine that you are a visitor from another planet, arriving on earth for the first time and exploring everything you can find. Your own planet would be at a different distance to the sun, so everything here appears bright and interesting. You would walk around the house and garden with a sense of pure fascination, observing colours, shapes and patterns, stillness and movement. Would you be able to make sense of the patterned wallpaper that remains unchanged, while the sunshine, shining through the window, makes continuous new patterns on the floor? Stand still and notice the sounds around you, and touch everything with a simple, naive fascination. Notice the textures of things and the hardness or softness; and like a toddler feel the temptation to put it to your lips. Notice the world from a brave new perspective.

OBSERVE YOURSELF

Taking the stance of the unprejudiced observer or the meta-observer, try watching yourself from the outside. This is not like looking at your own reflection in a mirror, but more a sort of stepping outside of yourself so that you notice your thoughts, feelings or body language as if they belong to someone else.

I was reduced to giggles in a large shopping centre, after doing this exercise for a few minutes. I don't like shopping centres myself, but I was with someone who wanted to take the time to enjoy both shopping and window shopping. I was getting more and more irritated and finally detached myself to rush through a department store to buy the one item I actually needed. I'm not sure what triggered my decision to try mindfulness while I was doing this, but suddenly the image came to me of, 'Irritable woman with a frown on her face, scurrying through a seemingly endless display of large, polished, expensive handbags.' There was something about the size and elegance of the handbags that felt completely foreign to my inner experience of impatience and irritability; so that I started to laugh. With laughter came self-compassion, and as my irritability dropped away I found that I could simply enjoy the shopping centre as if it was a museum of anthropology.

THREE-MINUTE MEDITATION

This is a quick meditation that is traditionally done in three minutes, but can be done in less. There are three steps to it. Step one is to sit or stand in an upright dignified posture with a straight back and eyes closed if that is comfortable for you. Bring your awareness to your inner experience and ask yourself, 'What is happening right now?' Notice what thoughts are in your mind, and what feelings you have. Accept any unpleasant experiences or negativity, without trying to change it. Notice any body sensations such as tension, discomfort or pain, but don't try and change them in any way.

Step two is to narrow your attention to one aspect of your breathing, such as the air going in through your nostrils, or your belly rising and falling with the rhythm of your breath. Keep in the present moment, observing your breath and when the mind wants to wander, gently bring it back.

Step three takes you back into an expanded awareness again. From focusing on the breath in step two, you can start breathing into the whole body. Notice any sensations or feelings in the body, and acknowledge them with a friendly curiosity, without trying to change them.

You could practise this as a three-minute refresher before the next patient arrives, sitting quietly in your practice chair. Feel your body being supported by the chair and quietly allow everything to slow down as you focus first on your body, then on your breathing and then back to your body again. Just witness yourself – a practitioner waiting quietly in the clinic room – without judgement or comment.

ONE-MINUTE MEDITATION: STOP THE TRAFFIC

My colleague, Judit Weegmann, suggested this meditation to me.

Sit quietly with both feet on the floor and close your eyes or look at something neutral like the carpet. Imagine you are an old-fashioned traffic policeman, the sort that wears white gloves to direct the traffic. You're standing at a complex road junction, perhaps on a raised podium like the conductor of an orchestra. The traffic rushes by you, until you turn towards one column of traffic, and hold up your hands in the universal signal that tells them to stop. All the vehicles come to a halt.

You might see the faces of the drivers – the anger or frustration that they had to stop, the wish to carry on going, even the attempt to drive through the 'red light'. You need to look at them with all the confidence of your authority and with your raised hands telling them they have to stop.

Then you turn to face the other column of traffic, hold up your hands and they stop as well. Now all is silent and still. Enjoy the stillness and peacefulness of the moment. Breathe quietly. Stay like this as long as you like it. No hurry. You feel the peace. Now it is not only you who is in peace standing in the middle of the silent traffic but all the drivers become peaceful as well. They have come to terms with your decision that they had to stop. They are looking at you in peace now. You are looking at them in peace and confidence. You are the judge of the situation about when the traffic will be ready to go again. They have accepted this as well.

When you're ready, choose which column you will let go first. This is your choice. You don't need to move just yet; just imagine which column will go first. Does it feel comfortable and right? If it doesn't, then change your mind and imagine that you will let the other column go. Does that feel comfortable? Change your mind as many times as you feel like it. It will not take too long. You will come to a comfortable decision within one minute. Don't worry about taking your time.

Once you feel okay about it, indicate that one column of traffic may start, and go in a certain direction. When you let them go they will start in a calm and peaceful manner.

You might enjoy watching them for a few seconds before you bring your meditation to a close.

Although it might seem as if this meditation takes a long time, be reassured that even in the most hectic times this meditation doesn't take more than a minute or two. You can do it two to three times a day to bring yourself back into a more neutral and quiet state of mind.

GETTING OFF THE TREADMILL

Relaxing the mind in this way, even if it is only for a few minutes, takes time out from the busyness of the day. It is the opposite of the continuous, mindless, unstructured chatter of the brain that can take up a needless amount of energy and creates unnecessary stress. Mindfulness cuts away the past and the future and allows you to just be in the present. This is the state that you wish to be in, when in consultation with a patient.

▋ REFLECTIVE EXAMPLE

For homework my tutor on the mindfulness training course said that we had to eat one meal a day mindfully. I immediately felt guilty, because even when I'm on my own I never just eat a meal – I'm either catching up on my reading or I'm checking something on my computer. So this morning I had my breakfast as mindfully as I could manage: an apple chopped up into muesli with plain yoghurt. I suppose I could have started the mindfulness at the preparation stage, but instead I started it when I sat down to eat.

I felt a pleasurable anticipation at sitting down to eat. It looked appetizing, and I could feel my digestive juices getting ready as I was quite hungry. The appearance of my breakfast satisfied me – no, more than that, it pleased me. The apple skin was red and the raisins were black against the white of the yoghurt. I normally eat fast so this time I tried to eat slowly and be aware of the food. The smell was cool and fresh, the taste was tangy and sharp and there was just the right amount of sweetness in the raisins. (I hate too much sweet stuff at breakfast.) I noticed that as I ate, I favoured one side of my mouth. I wonder why that is? Does it date back to a painful tooth in the past?

What really surprised me was the noise! I had no idea that eating was so noisy. There was the crashing of my spoon against the bowl, the crunch of the apple, the sounds of chewing and swallowing: it was all so loud! Even with my cup of tea I sounded as if I was gulping it down.

I didn't find it easy. It sounded easy when the tutor told us to do it, but keeping my focus on simply eating, when I wanted to think about the movie I saw last night and what I needed to do for the rest of the day… I kept having to pull my attention back to my breakfast. I realized how easy it was to tune out from what I was doing (feeding myself, nourishing myself) even to the point of not hearing all of that noise because I was overfamiliar with it. It makes me wonder if my mind is always somewhere else than with what I'm actually doing.

I wonder if there have been times when I have eaten with full appreciation of the here and now? One circumstance that comes to mind is when we have been hillwalking or fell walking, we choose a high viewpoint where we will stop for lunch. The climb up to the viewpoint is always steep and the going is tough, so that by the time we sit down and admire the view my limbs are tired but my spirit is exalting. I sit and look over my view and feel incredibly happy and satisfied. I don't feel the need to think about anything. I'm empty after the exertion of my walk. I am just there. The roughly put-together sandwich of bread and cheese with a cherry tomato tastes absolutely delicious. I am on top of the world.

It would be good to get something near that state when I am eating at home. Over the next few days, if the weather is good, I think I will experiment with having my lunch sitting on my balcony in a mindful way.

EXERCISE: SELF-COMPASSION

Divide your page into three columns. In the first column, write down your experiences of the first few cases that you took at the beginning of your career. You can be ruthless and include things that you forgot to do or did badly. In the last column, write down all of the characteristics you imagine a perfect practitioner would have. In the middle column, make an assessment of where you are now, somewhere between your fumbling beginnings as a practitioner, and the perfect ideal. Now tell yourself in your own words, or read my words aloud:

'I will always be in the middle column, gradually moving away from awkwardness and anxiety, towards perfection. I won't ever reach the final column of perfection, but it doesn't matter. I can be good enough, and that will be fine for my patients. From now on I'm going to be the good-enough practitioner, always improving little by little, always developing, always expanding, always exploring, always moving forwards, never getting there. It's as if the goalposts are always moving or the horizon is always expanding. That is the way of the world and it's okay. I feel quite excited knowing that my practice will never be static, I will always be learning and developing. It feels okay to know that I'll never be perfect and I don't have to be perfect. I like the thought that all practitioners are in the same position, even those practitioners that I admire greatly as experts and teachers. All of us are moving forward at our own pace, and that fills me with a sort of relief. I can take my time to enjoy where I am now without always looking where I have been or where I want to go. All is well.'

EXERCISE: MINDFULNESS MEDITATION

Choose a small object that has meaning for you from your desk, briefcase, bag or rucksack. Sit on the floor with your legs crossed, or sit in a seat with your feet flat on the floor, and hold your chosen object loosely in your lap. If it is restful for you, close your eyes. Rock a couple of times on your sitting bones to make yourself more comfortable. Concentrate on your breathing and increase your awareness of the breath going in and out of your lungs and nose. As you exhale, relax the little muscles around your face and neck. Take one deeper inhalation and let it out in a sigh. Then allow your breathing to return to normal. Take a few minutes to just sit and enjoy breathing.

Become aware of the sounds around you. Can you hear the sounds of your own breathing, other people in the building, animals or children outside, or the sounds of vehicles or aeroplanes? Try to be totally aware of the sounds as if you're immersed in them, as if you are just a pair of ears and nothing else. Don't think or analyse too much, just live with the sounds from minute to minute.

Keeping your eyes shut, start to explore your special object, gently touching it with your fingertips. Try not to analyse what you feel, but like a child simply enjoy the sensory experience of its shape, texture, softness, hardness, heat, cold, rigidity or flexibility. If you want, you can raise it to your face and touch it against your lips or stroke it against your cheek. If it is appropriate, touch it against your tongue to taste it. Try not to analyse or think about it, and if any memories arise around it, tell yourself that you will think about these later.

Raise your object to your nose and breathe deeply. Don't try to analyse any smells that you notice. Just become involved in receiving the smells.

Finally, open your eyes and take your time to look at your object. Turn it around slowly, so that you can see it from different angles, and appreciate its shape, its design, its colour and its texture. See it as if for the first time, with a calm, objective, gentle curiosity.

When you're ready, slowly come back to the present, and write notes about what you experienced.

EXERCISE: APPRECIATING MINDFULLY

Choose something from your environment that you can observe with care and appreciate in detail. Have you ever held a tender, young holly leaf in the palm of your hand and observed with wonderment the reddish, almost translucent tinge to the leaf – the silky, slippery, flexible feel of it – and the soft, bendy spines that don't prickle at all? Have you ever watched a butterfly dancing its way through the soft summer breezes and landing almost as if by surprise on a flower, its wings fluttering like delicate petals, as timelessly beautiful as the flower itself?

Take the time to give something your full, unprejudiced and appreciative attention without presupposing outcomes or remembering previous similar occasions; just simply appreciating it for what it is.

Chapter 6

SKILLS FOR CASE-TAKING

Many patients prepare their story in advance of visiting an alternative practitioner. This is probably the same story that they have been telling themselves as well as telling friends, family and various practitioners. It is a narrative that includes their present symptoms, the history of the complaint, a probable diagnosis as well as some of their fears and anxieties about being unwell. Often the narrative is slightly distorted or exaggerated, whether intentionally or not. If it is exaggerated, it might be deliberate in order to get a speedy treatment – which is a fair tactic on behalf of the patient. If it is distorted, symptoms might be misrepresented according to their emotional significance; things that are feared can be exaggerated or glossed over.

The story narrative has to be abbreviated when visiting a GP (general practitioner) due to time restraints, while the alternative practitioner who has more time, is usually given a longer version. It always needs further exploration to clarify details and uncover missing elements. It is only the first level of truth which is masking another, deeper story. When the caring practitioner takes time to ensure that the patient feels safe and respected and listens attentively, the layers can be peeled back to reveal a fuller story.

HOMEOPATHIC CASE-TAKING

Of all the alternative therapies, homeopathy involves the most in-depth case-taking, so homeopaths need highly developed questioning and listening skills similar to those of a PCA (person-centred approach) counsellor. The first appointment usually lasts an hour and a half or longer, and 30–45 minutes for the follow-ups. This chapter was written with homeopaths in mind, encouraging them to take the fullest possible case so that they can understand their patient on mental, emotional and physical levels. Practitioners with therapies that divide the first session into case-taking and an initial treatment will obviously have less time for in-depth case-taking, and can cherry pick through the information offered here.

Ian Townsend (2011) has been studying the parallels between homeopathy and person-centred counselling (PCA). He has listed 20 points of similarity between them and concludes, 'the similarities between the philosophy, theory, and *in-the-consulting-room* practice of our two disciplines are remarkably striking' (p.19).

Homeopathy is not a talk therapy as such, but the practitioner needs to understand the patient as thoroughly as possible in order to make an accurate prescription. Homeopathic philosophy is based upon *like cures like*. This means that remedy descriptions must match the patient's symptoms *and* their emotional characteristics in order for them to be effective. Even if the presenting symptoms are physical, the homeopath still needs a holistic picture, so they encourage the patient to talk about their moods and feelings as well. It is not the intention of the homeopath to become a lay counsellor or psychotherapist. However the similar questioning techniques and the quiet, warm, compassionate attention of the practitioner encourage the patient to talk freely about themselves.

The difference between homeopathy and PCA counselling is in the homeopathic prescription which can leapfrog the patient into mental, emotional or physical healing, much faster than weekly counselling. If there is a placebo effect it would be noted equally by both therapies. The following sentence by Townsend (2011) can apply to many alternative therapies:

> The primacy given to each client's narrating of her own story to an unprejudiced observer... who can through active listening, mirroring, checking out/reflecting back, and empathic (? shamanic) processes, work with/at the edge of awareness whilst equally valuing all configurations of self (symptom pattern matching) at the same time being true to and aware of own self (congruence, self-awareness) in other words, acknowledging the importance of the therapeutic relationship. (p.22)

It is worth taking the time to unpack this. Townsend begins this sentence with the patient being given the freedom to tell her story narrative to a practitioner who is unprejudiced. Various skills are employed to enable the patient to talk freely, such as active listening, mirroring and checking out/reflecting back. (All discussed later in this chapter.) Practitioner empathy is necessary so that these skills can be used effectively. Beyond that there is the willingness to risk working at the edge of awareness which will possibly result in transformation. All aspects of the patient's being are acknowledged and valued by the practitioner, who continues to be aware of their own self and remain true to themselves. The importance of the therapeutic relationship is at the heart of both therapies.

Working at the edge of awareness is to work on unstable ground. It gives the patient the space to uncover the unknown and through this new understanding, make great changes to their life. But if the patient is uncovering the unknown, then the same will be happening to you, the practitioner. In order to work this way, you need to have a commitment towards your own journey of self-discovery.

IN THE CONSULTING ROOM

The aim of the practitioner from any pathway, whether you are alternative or traditional, is to get the information you need during the consultation in order to form a treatment plan. The worst scenario is when a practitioner doesn't have enough time and has to rush through a question and answer routine, with little consideration for the patient. Then the direct questions only give room for yes or no answers, and the patient feels dissatisfied because they have not explained themselves properly. They will probably feel that a hasty practitioner lacks respect, care, genuineness, or kindness. At its worst, a tin-opener consultation will leave the patient feeling emotionally invaded, and the discerning patient will not return to that practitioner if they can help it.

On the other hand, the compassionate practitioner balances support and encouragement with challenges that are tactful and appropriate. Support and encouragement are necessary because the patient is vulnerable and exposed while telling their story. When you use tactful and appropriate challenges, you encourage the patient to dig deeper and give more information. You will be consciously balancing the intention of loving kindness towards the patient with pushing them to reveal themselves. You do this proactively through carefully worded questions, active listening and open body language. You also do it reactively, using non-verbal sounds (such as 'mmm'), empathetic facial expressions and focused body language.

QUESTIONING SKILLS: GETTING THE PATIENT TO SAY MORE

The patient has arrived, and has had their physiological needs and their safety needs satisfied. You have introduced yourself and negotiated a working agreement. Before inviting the patient to tell their narrative story, you should briefly signpost what will happen throughout the rest of the consultation, explaining how the time will be spent from now on, either in case-taking or in active treatment.

Once you have invited the patient to begin their narrative story, you should sit quietly and just listen until the patient has finished talking. Your body language, facial expression and non-verbal noises ('mmm') will show your interest. Some people talk about their personal issues easily, while others need a lot of encouragement. The really loquacious patient might need interrupting if they digress and start talking about someone else's problems. The shy and hesitant patient might need extra non-verbal encouragement with your smiles and nods.

When the patient has had their say, you can ask them to tell you more about the main issue (see Box 6.1). The best way to do this is using open questions. These are non-directive and open-ended questions, allowing the patient the freedom to answer in any way they want, such as: 'How do you feel about that?', 'Describe that to me', 'Tell me about your appetite', 'How is your sleep?' Open questions give the patient permission to tell their story as fully as possible and give you time to feel the patient's presence as well as listen to them.

BOX 6.1 QUESTIONING TECHNIQUES

- Open questions
- Closed questions
- Asking, 'Tell me more'
- Echoing their words (parroting)
- Paraphrasing
- Conjecturing

The opposite of open questions are closed questions, which invite yes or no answers, such as, 'Do you have a good appetite?' or 'Do you sleep well?' These limit the patient and have a certain hit-and-miss quality that demands a lot of effort on your part with minimum results. The patient is left feeling frustrated if their specific issues are not mentioned among the questions; or they become passive assuming you know best. However, there are times when closed questions are necessary. For instance, as the consultation draws towards the finish, you can ask more closed questions to clarify the details of earlier statements.

There are other techniques that you can use to facilitate the patient to talk further, taking them to deeper levels where they reveal more about themselves. Sometimes you can just ask, 'Tell me more?' Echoing, sometimes called parroting, is the practice of repeating one or a few of the patient's words back to them again, with the spoken or implied question, 'Tell me more about this.' This is quite straightforward when it refers to physical symptoms, like 'Tell me more about your nausea.' or 'Tell me more about your headaches.' If you want to find out more about their moods and feelings, a question could be as simple as, 'You said you feel anxious when you're driving?' Your tone of voice will turn this into a question. Echoing the patient's words back to them encourages them to really explore what they mean and uncover deeper meaning.

Sometimes it is less obvious which keyword to echo to gain revealing information from the patient. Take note of any dissonance between the words spoken and the body language or facial expression, like the patient who says they are doing well, while quickly wiping a watery eye. You could echo back the words, 'Doing well?'

Other anomalies might be the unintentional emphasis, an uncharacteristic swear word or the hesitation in an otherwise smooth delivery. You can echo any of these back to the patient as a way of getting them to talk more about the subject. One of my patients, an upright, middle-class, churchgoing woman in her 40s came to me for re-occurring cystitis. When I asked her to describe the cystitis, we were both startled by her unexpected usage of coarse language. She put her hand over her mouth and apologized; but I reassured her. It gave me a great insight into what remedy she might need.

Sudden changes in the hand gestures, the body language, the tone or volume of speech might all be worth investigating. Sometimes it is appropriate to mirror the patient's body language, which shows empathy and could give you an insight into how the patient is feeling. Sometimes it is useful to tell the patient what you noticed about their body language saying, 'You were doing…with your hands when you said that.' This might be rotating their hands, stroking them, clenching them or sitting on them. Bringing this unconscious gesture into the patient's viewpoint can open up the case. It also facilitates the patient's own understanding of themselves.

Paraphrasing, sometimes called active listening, usually works with a larger quantity of information. Rather than repeating back a single word or short phrase as you would when echoing, you repeat a larger chunk of information in your own words, in order to double-check your understanding and reassure the patient that you are listening. One practitioner always begins paraphrasing with the kindly, avuncular phrase, 'Let me understand you…' Another might say, 'So your pains seem to get worse during the night, and are definitely worse first thing in the morning, but they get much better once you start moving. Am I correct?'

Conjecturing is a form of tentative conclusion that you offer in such a way that the patient can accept, reject or add to the information. Conjectures begin with slightly hesitant phrases such as, 'I was wondering if…', 'One possibility is…' or 'It occurred to me that…' The implication is that this is just a suggestion that might or might not help the patient's explanation of the problem. It can trigger further thoughts or descriptions from the patient. Another advantage of conjectures is that they reassure the patient that you are thinking about the case without jumping to conclusions.

A less hesitant form of the conjecture, is to make a statement and invite the patient's response as to whether this fits the case, such as, 'Your stomach upsets and constipation seem to be directly linked to eating rich food and drinking alcohol.' Your facial expression and hand gestures invite feedback to the statement.

You might find that the most difficult task is to wait in silence while the patient is thinking through their answer. If you are impatient you might want to help the patient along by offering multiple choice questions. These might elicit some sort of answer, but doing this can make the patient divert from the answer they were reaching for. It is far better to wait, while watching the patient's body language so as to not interrupt their thought processes. Neighbour (2005) writes about the 'internal search':

The attention is directed inwards while thoughts and memories begin to associate in the imagination. The body becomes relatively still; the eyes become defocused, and sometimes move rapidly as they scan the images projected in the mind's eye. Almost invariably the end result of this internal search is something significant – a new insight, or a relevant memory, or a possible link between two previously unrelated ideas. (p.157)

You should train yourself to wait in non-verbal attentive silence until the patient's body becomes less still, they move or relax the shoulders and the eyes become more focused, perhaps resuming eye contact again. They are then ready to resume dialogue and if encouraged, they will reveal their thoughts or new understanding. When working with students, I ask them to do a role-play in which one of them is the storyteller and one is the case-taker. The case-taker has to ask an opening question, such as, 'Tell me about your summer holidays.' After that they are allowed just two more questions and will have to rely on their non-verbal communication skills to keep the storyteller talking for ten minutes. It is an interesting exercise as it forces them to stop talking and concentrate on other communication skills.

LISTENING SKILLS: THE GIFT OF BEING QUIET

Hearing is the function of the ears which automatically sense the vibrations of sound. Listening is the conscious choice to focus on and understand what is being heard, and it can be done with greater or lesser commitment and concentration.

Imagine a sliding scale, with being totally present for the patient at the top end of the scale and being oblivious to the patient at the other end. Most practitioners fall somewhere in the middle. An experienced practitioner can listen whole-heartedly, taking the minimum of notes on automatic pilot. For a student or inexperienced practitioner, a larger amount of concentration goes into the note-taking, detracting from the listening. The ability to listen carefully becomes even more diminished when they are trying to make a clinical diagnosis and treatment plan at the same time, or they are planning their answer or their feedback. Further down the scale is when the practitioner's inner voice starts talking, introducing prejudices, criticisms or comparisons with the self, and at the bottom of the scale is the appearance of empathic listening while their mind is engaged in personal issues.

BOX 6.2 HOW CLOSELY DO YOU LISTEN?

- Listening with empathy and being totally present
- Listening to the story and making notes
- Listening while thinking of an answer or making a clinical diagnosis
- Listening divided between what the patient says and your own thoughts
- Appearing to listen but actually miles away thinking of personal issues

---

The different levels of listening can be seen in the body language. For example, if you watch two or three people casually chatting together, their body language is relaxed, they change position easily, they give the speaker sufficient eye contact, but feel free to look away and they might even give quick scans around the room. It is clear that their concentration is divided between their personal issues, their thoughts about how they can contribute to the conversation, and listening to the speaker.

On the other hand when the listener decides to give their full concentration to the speaker, there is a change in body language that denotes empathy. The listener becomes more still and focused and they engage with more eye contact, although this varies with different cultures. They will probably move closer to the speaker and might match their body language or point knees, feet or hands towards them. Small changes of facial expression show that the listener is following both the facts of the story and the underlying emotions. They might make small non-verbal noises such as, 'ah' or 'mmm' as well as giving explicit nods or shakes of the head. There might be changes in the listener's breathing such as holding the breath or sighing.

It is this level of empathic listening that the patient craves and the caring practitioner aims towards. It demonstrates that you are walking alongside the patient, understanding their journey step-by-step. Carl Rogers (1961) wrote in *On Becoming a Person*:

> This kind of sensitive, active listening is exceedingly rare in our lives. We think we listen, but very rarely do we listen with real understanding, true empathy. Yet listening, of this very special kind, is one of the most potent forces for change that I know. (pp.115–116)

Active listening benefits both you and your patient. For you, it is a decision to do less rather than more, to empty your mind of unnecessary thoughts and just be with the patient. This is mindful listening, engaging in the here and now, without reference to what has been or will be. For the patient, it is the opportunity to listen to themselves, to identify and refine their thoughts and feelings about their symptoms. It builds up their trust in you and enables them to speak about things that they rarely or never speak about. Often these issues are at the heart of the case.

If you're busy as a practitioner you might argue that there isn't enough time within the consultation to just sit and listen. However, Youngson (2012) suggests that time seems to expand when the mind is still:

> The first step in finding time to care is simply to stop. Give your patient complete attention. Bring stillness to your mind and be attentive to what is happening. Magic happens in these precious moments.
>
> In our clockwork analogy of the Universe, we have an idea of time as something rigid, punctuated and inflexible. This sense of time is reinforced when our care becomes nothing more than a series of tasks. When care is mechanical, time becomes rigid.
>
> But the human experience of time is quite different. In moments of close connection, time stands still. Research shows that patients who attend a doctor skilled in interpersonal connection believe their appointment was much longer than the allocated time. (p.132)

When you take the time to really listen to the patient, you contribute to the level four on Maslow's hierarchy of needs, the level of self-esteem, confidence, self-respect and respect by others. This is the deepest acknowledgement of the patient by the practitioner. It opens them up to the possibility of healing.

OBSERVATION SKILLS: WORKING WITH
NON-VERBAL COMMUNICATION

Samuel Hahnemann (1810) writing in *The Organon* stressed the importance of objective observation of the patient, as opposed to speculating what might be wrong:

> Aphorism 6: The unprejudiced observer realizes the futility of metaphysical speculations that cannot be verified by experiment, and no matter how clever he is, he sees in any given case of disease only the disturbances of body and soul which are perceptible to the senses: subjective symptoms, incidental symptoms, objective symptoms, i.e., deviations from the former healthy condition of the individual now sick which the patient personally feels, which people around him notice, which the physician sees in him. (p.11)

This is even more important when we consider that the larger percentage of communication is acted out on a non-verbal level, through the body language, facial expression, gestures, changes in the voice and autonomic responses such as the breathing. Your body language, including your posture and the position on your seat can express confidence in an open, more exposed body posture, or lack of confidence in a closed, guarded position (see Figure 6.1). Your feet or knees frequently point in the direction that you are interested in. Your hand gestures and facial expressions can change from minute to minute. When your hand strokes your chin, it can be a thinking gesture, as long as your hand doesn't take the weight of the whole head which can mean boredom. Your voice can vary in tone, rhythm, pitch or intensity, slowing down as you become more thoughtful (or tired) and speeding up with excitement or fear. Autonomic responses such as changes in your breathing patterns or blushing can also happen.

Much of non-verbal communication happens automatically and is beyond conscious awareness. In many situations we understand and react to other people's non-verbal signals without knowing why. We say, 'I had a gut feeling.'

You can use your own body language to smooth the pathway of the consultation and reassure the patient. This is because most people unconsciously copy or mirror another's hand gestures, facial expressions or tone of voice. If you deliberately sit with a relaxed, open but not overly confident body language you're creating a posture which the patient will unconsciously copy. The uptight patient in front of you will relax and become more open themselves.

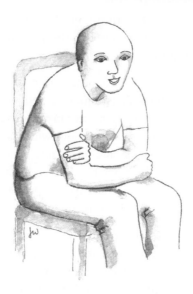

FIGURE 6.1: OBSERVE THE PATIENT'S BODY LANGUAGE

If you increase your awareness of non-verbal communication, you can understand your patients on a deeper level. The more subtle nuances of body language and facial expression are extremely difficult to fake, especially when someone is talking at the same time. When you are observing carefully, you are more likely to notice anomalies when a patient's words say one thing while their body language says something else. I was sitting in a cafe one day having lunch and amusing myself with people-watching via some large tilted mirrors that lined the walls. A young man was dreamily watching two girls at another table, and out of curiosity I turned to look directly at his feet to see which girl he was interested in, as his feet would point towards her. But his feet had a life of their own and they were stretching towards the handbag that one of them had thrown on the floor, ready to drag it towards him. Startled, I said to the girl, 'Watch out for your handbag!' She grabbed it quickly and the would-be thief swore at me and strode out of the cafe.

While you are observing the patient, the patient will be just as eagerly observing you, noticing everything consciously or unconsciously. They will notice things like the warmth of your welcome, your smile, whether your body language is welcoming, whether your tone of voice shows you're taking them seriously and whether you're looking at your computer or notes more than you look at them. It is all carefully observed, often unconsciously, in order to assess whether you are a nice person and trustworthy.

Mirror neurons in the brain cause us to recreate another's emotion just by watching them. It is an inbuilt capacity that enables children to mimic their parents, siblings and other carers in order to learn; and it remains with us throughout our lives. In *Help for the Helper: A Psychophysiology of Compassion Fatigue and Vicarious Trauma*, Babette Rothschild (2006) writes:

> Adopting a particular facial expression will communicate emotional information to the brain. The same process is involved whether the facial expression is generated inside you or is set in motion by copying the expression of another. (p.76)

Postural mirroring, as it is called, happens unconsciously all the time and includes the imitation of someone else's physical posture and facial expressions. These in turn, inform the emotions of the observer. The way it plays out is something like this: one person feels the emotion, which is simultaneously expressed physically through their facial expressions and body language. The other person automatically imitates these physical stances which immediately recreates the feeling or emotion in them. When this is looked at with reference to the practitioner–patient relationship, the ramifications are many.

If the patient has strong emotions, you can pick these up through mirroring the patient's body language or facial expression and then feeling the emotions. In the short term this enables you to feel empathy and to show this to the patient. However, if you do this a lot and do it subconsciously without acknowledging that you copied the body language from your patient, you might find the patient's emotions stay with you after the patient has left. (More about this in Chapter 12.)

On the other hand, copying the patient's body language can have its advantages. If you want to reflect further on your patient after the session, or you have taken the case to a supervisor, one way is to mime them. Sitting, moving, and gesturing as if you are your patient, enables you to get under the skin of the patient and understand them from inside out. However, you do need to back up your insights with further analysis.

OBSERVE YOURSELF: YOU ARE PART OF THE DYNAMIC

Sometimes it is very useful to observe your own thoughts, emotions or bodily sensations, when you're working with one of your patients. Some patients are a delight to work with. They talk easily or have a sense of humour; they remember all of your instructions and advice and give you regular feedback after each prescription or treatment. Other patients are slow to get well, depressing to talk to, miss appointments or forget to follow your instructions. In these cases it is unsurprising that you should look forward to one patient and feel a heart-sink at the other.

A simple way of testing how you feel about a patient, is to note your mood when you see their name in the appointments book or receive a text or an e-mail from them. Once you have identified that you have negative feelings about a patient, you can then do some work in your reflective journal to explore why you feel like that. It might be because they remind you of someone else – or remind you of some less attractive aspect of yourself. These patients provide the perfect opportunity for you to get to understand yourself, and progress with your self-development.

When you are in clinic with patients, it can be helpful to take note of any reactions in your body to their story. My own experience is that when facing a new patient who holds a lot of grief, I would start to feel tight and congested in my upper chest or throat, as if I was feeling their grief. As I'm generally a happy person and don't hold a lot of grief, I would take this as a sign that my body was mirroring theirs. The feeling went as soon as we started talking, but it was a useful warning of what to look out for. If I had the sensation of tightness or any other bodily feeling after the patient has left, I would do some self-reflection about where this came from, and what to do about it. See Chapter 9 on boundaries for more about this.

EFFECTIVE CASE-TAKING

Your case-taking underpins both your on-going relationship with the patient and your treatment plan for the current session. To make your case-taking effective, you need to have an attitude of curiosity, interest, respect and compassion; and you need to have understood and practised the skills of listening, questioning and observing.

Case-taking is not an exact science. We can rationalize the different types of questioning techniques, but how a question is delivered is as important as the content, especially when both you and the patient are observing each other's non-verbal clues. In Townsend's (2011) words, the practitioner is always 'working at the edge of awareness' (p.22) with the patient, trying to understand them and perhaps, enable them to understand themselves.

REFLECTIVE EXAMPLE

My supervisor asked me to audit my listening skills for a week. I have decided to audit the following criteria:

- appropriate eye contact according to the other person's needs
- being aurally present for the other person without listening to my inner thoughts
- waiting in silence
- encouraging with open body language
- non-verbal sounds like 'hmm' and 'ah'.

I can see that waiting in silence will be difficult for me, without finishing the other person's sentence or asking them twenty questions to help them along.

Day one

My patient in clinic was quite elderly and hard of hearing. Case-taking was slow, and I felt I needed to exaggerate some of my listening skills because of her deficiency. My eye contact was slightly longer than usual, my non-verbal sounds were louder and my body language was exaggerated. The patient took so long to answer some of the questions that I did try to help her out by suggesting answers, so I wasn't good at waiting in silence. (But can I justify myself by saying this was appropriate? Probably not.) As for being aurally present, I think I was in hyperdrive with my own thoughts while she was thinking so slowly. All in all, not a very good example of attentive listening skills.

Day two

My patient in clinic was much younger than yesterday's and I felt I had a good connection with her, dividing my attention between eye contact and looking down at my notes so that she didn't feel stared at. I spent five minutes sitting quietly before she arrived, to calm my mind and empty some of my stuff, so I felt I was quite present for her. I found I could wait in silence, but she didn't keep me waiting too long as most of her answers came easily to her. I started off with deliberately open body language, and about halfway through I noticed that I was mirroring some of her body language. I was pleased about this as it showed empathy. I think I used a lot of non-verbal sounds.

Day three

There was no one booked into clinic, so I audited listening to my good friend. The first noticeable differences between my friend and a patient were that we sat much closer together, touched each other at times and had more eye contact. I had no time to prepare myself, like I did yesterday, as she launched immediately into telling me about her weekend. I found my attention changed at different points in her story. Sometimes I was totally with her, and at other times my own thoughts took over, comparing her experiences with my own. So I did miss some of her story. What really pleased me however, was that I managed to listen in silence and I didn't finish one sentence for her. More than once, I opened my mouth to speak and then remembered to shut up or say softly, 'mmm'? I felt quite proud of myself by the end, and I asked my friend if she had noticed. She said she had felt less hurried by me. I hadn't realized that my habit of interrupting silence made anyone feel hurried.

Day four

My patient in clinic was a young girl who was very shy and quietly spoken. I found myself automatically copying her in using a soft voice, and I decided to give her less eye contact than I would normally. I deliberately make my body language open and reminded myself, 'No interrupting.' It was very tough, as I really, really wanted to help her along by giving multiple-choice questions and had to force myself into just using non-verbal sounds and gentle smiles. To my surprise, it worked and she began to open up and say more. I found I had so much to do with giving her non-verbal feedback, that I was totally present.

Day five

No patients again so I decided to practise my listening skills on my nephew. He is aged four and adorable. Usually we both speak at the same time, along with a lot of cuddling and wrestling. This time we didn't have much eye contact because he was sitting on my lap but we had body contact instead. After working on it all week I found I could just listen to him without talking, with only one or two lapses. To my surprise, when I really listened to him, there was much less wriggling and wrestling. His body language became much calmer, and I felt much more present.

Conclusions

It's been a really interesting exercise to consciously practise good listening skills and record the results. I found some things like eye contact and body language varied according to the other person's needs. The rest was up to me deliberately controlling my urge to talk and using more non-verbal skills such as facial expression and making small sounds. It gave me quite a shock when my friend said that my interruptions had made her feel hurried; and I was very surprised when my nephew was calmer without all my talking. These have been big lessons for me, showing me that learning to keep quiet will benefit everyone else and in time I will benefit, too.

EXERCISE: QUESTIONING SKILLS

Watch a TV interview between a proficient interviewer and a celebrity. Jot down what type of questions are used, such as open or closed questions or echoing. Make a note of which type of questions are effective.

To take this further, notice how the interviewer behaves. What is their body language? Do they have an aggressive interviewing style or a friendly one? Do they let the interviewee give non-answers or do they push hard to get the answer they want?

EXERCISE: QUESTIONING SKILLS

Imagine you are taking the case of a new patient or client, as an alternative practitioner (choose your own therapy). The challenge is that you need to take a full case, but you're only allowed six different questions, which you can repeat as many times as you like. What would your six questions be? Write them down into your reflective journal, and review them after two to three weeks to see if you still agree with your original thoughts.

EXERCISE: LISTENING SKILLS

The next time a family member or friend wants to tell you something, stop what else you are doing and listen with full attention and empathy. Afterwards make some notes in your journal about what it felt like for you as listener and whether you noticed any difference in the speaker's delivery.

EXERCISE: LISTENING SKILLS

Arrange with a colleague or friend to practise your listening skills. Ask them about their holidays as a child and listen with full attention and empathy. Try listening in complete silence, or allow yourself to ask one question only. Afterwards make some notes in your journal about what it felt like for you as a listener, and get feedback on the experience from the other person.

EXERCISE: OBSERVATIONAL SKILLS

Get a good book on body language (such as the books by Allan Pease) and – if you can do it unobtrusively – practise your people-watching on the train or in a supermarket. See what you can read from their body language, gestures and facial expressions.

EXERCISE: OBSERVATIONAL SKILLS

Increase your awareness of your own mirror neurons. While watching a movie, notice how many times you smile in reaction to an actor smiling, or weep as the actor weeps. Notice the little twitches of your own muscles in response to the actor shrugging their shoulders, clenching their fists, kicking a ball, or any other physical activity.

Chapter 7

REDUCING YOUR PREJUDICES AND LIMITING BELIEFS

Prejudice about other people and limiting beliefs about yourself amount to the same thing: a narrowed horizon and low expectations arising from fixed opinions that haven't been properly thought through. Limiting beliefs are about yourself and can be about your health, wealth, gender, age, ability to achieve, position in society, education and so on. Prejudice is about people other than you, and can be about gender, race, colour, sexuality, age, religion, socio-economic status and so on. These fixed beliefs can come from personal experience or be passed down from previous generations and become integrated into the family or the community as facts.

The disadvantages of bringing prejudices or limiting beliefs into the consulting room are many, for instance:

- low expectations for the patient's health and welfare

- low expectations of the practitioner's ability to help

- inability to see the patient as they really are and take the case fairly

- tendency to blame the patient for any failure in communication

- ascendancy of the practitioner's self-justifier (It's not my fault!)

- favouritism towards one treatment regime over another, regardless of what would suit the patient

- hesitation towards self-improvement or continuing professional development

- further loss of self-confidence.

When you are carrying prejudices or limiting beliefs they inhibit the flow of the consultation. It is more difficult to be completely present in a mindful way when you're with the patient. Your compassion can easily be blocked by prejudice about the patient or limiting beliefs about yourself.

LIMITING BELIEFS

Limiting beliefs are negative thought patterns that you have continued to repeat to yourself over time. They are the negative stories you tell yourself about yourself. They are a habit of thinking that is often deeply rooted and such a familiar part of your thinking that you are unaware of them. They limit your opportunities because they are continuously telling you that you are less than capable or you are not worthy of success. They feed off any underlying fear, depression, doubt, overwhelm, pessimism or other negative emotions.

If you're reading this, thinking that you don't have any limiting beliefs, a quick way to check is to ask yourself to finish this sentence: 'I'm no good at...' Don't be surprised if you immediately start to self-justify, such as you haven't had the time, money or opportunity. Saying you're no good at something is not the same as saying you have never studied it and have no knowledge of it. The expression 'no good' implies you have tried and failed. The difference is between saying, 'I've never properly studied another language apart from those two years at school,' and 'I failed my French exams for two years at school, therefore I'm hopeless with all languages.'

Some limiting beliefs come with an automatic self-justification, such as, 'I'm no good at...because of my...' Followed by something like your age, gender, health, education, and so on. This sort of belief comes with its own ball and chain, preventing you from even trying. A student in one of my university classes felt that her youth would hold her back in building a successful acupuncture practice. She was just out of school while many of her university classmates were mature students. They had life experience while she had study skills. She loved studying acupuncture but as she entered her third year she couldn't imagine herself as a practitioner treating someone older than herself. She felt she wouldn't get any respect from patients and they wouldn't listen to her advice, because she was so young. I asked her to reflect on whether the theme of being 'too young' had arisen at other times in her life, and I suggested that she asked her current, older classmates what qualities they thought she had as a practitioner.

Where do limiting beliefs come from? Writing in *The Biology of Belief: Unleashing the Power of Consciousness, Matter and Miracles*, Bruce Lipton (2005) explains:

> Young children carefully observe their environment and download the worldly wisdom offered by parents directly into their subconscious memory. As a result, their parents' behaviour and beliefs become their own. (p.133)

> The conscious mind is the creative one, the one that can conjure up 'positive thoughts.' In contrast, the subconscious mind is a repository of stimulus-response tapes derived from instincts and learned experiences. The subconscious mind is strictly habitual; it will play the same behavioural responses to life signals over and over again, much to our chagrin. (p.97)

When practitioners have limiting beliefs they can easily sabotage their own success. Many alternative practitioners learn their therapy for the sheer joy of it, but graduate with a scanty understanding of how to set up in practice. They can be further hampered by preconceptions that they are no good at business skills like advertising, networking, computer skills, giving public talks, explaining their therapy or doing their accounts. These limiting beliefs severely constrain the growth of the practice.

A limiting belief is a thought that you keep thinking, a conviction that is reinforced every time you think it or say it. However, the good news is you don't have to keep it. You can reframe it at any time. Some people like to do this abruptly by turning 180° and looking in the opposite direction. It is as if they suddenly become tired of always labelling themselves 'not good enough' at something and decide to gain some expertise in the subject. Sometimes events overtake you and you just have to learn the new skill. It happens to first-time parents, people who move house, those who start a new job, etc. They just have to dive in and learn new skills, feeling the fear and doing it anyway.

Not every limiting belief can be overturned easily and some are very deeply rooted, but it is still worthwhile taking the time to acknowledge it and working to diminish it. Sometimes it is possible to trace back to the beginning of that belief and ask questions. What was happening at the time? How old were you? What was the relevance of your original belief? Why do you think you locked this belief into place? Be compassionate towards yourself. You did the best you could at the time, considering what else was in the mix. Congratulate yourself that you now have the awareness and the tools to start dismantling the outdated belief.

My fixed belief that I was no good at sport or exercise began when I was about eight or nine. Prior to that I was invincible. Then I realized I was no good at PE or netball; I kept making mistakes, the other children laughed at me and I wasn't chosen by team leaders. What I didn't take into account was that my teacher always took off my glasses when we did any form of exercise, so I couldn't see what was happening. My negative experiences gradually consolidated into a limiting belief that I was no good at keeping fit, so for many years I stopped trying.

Even if you can't see the origin of your limiting belief, you can still begin to dismantle it by questioning its validity. This is best done using your reflective journal. Start off by writing your sentence beginning, 'I'm no good at…' Then put yourself into the role of the unprejudiced observer or the Leveller and ask yourself, 'Is it true?' Follow this by writing a list in your journal of all the times that you have been effective in some small way within the scope of your limiting belief. When you have finished, ask yourself again if you're really so deficient in that skill or knowledge. For example, I could write, 'I'm no good at getting exercise and keeping fit.' Then I would ask if it was true and list all of the times that I did get exercise, such as walking to work, walking up staircases rather than take the lift, carrying a heavy rucksack when I went on holiday or playing football with my nephew. I might find myself wanting to justify, such as, 'I only walk up the stairs at work because the lifts are overcrowded.' However, a few moments of reflection will show me that this still counts as exercise even if it was unintentional.

You could reflect further on your limiting beliefs by asking yourself the questions used by Byron Katie (2002) in her book, *Loving What Is: Four Questions That Can Change Your Life*:

- Is it true?

- Can you absolutely know that it's true?

- How do you react when you think that thought?

- Who would you be without the thought?

Byron Katie (2002) developed The Work as a system of inquiry into limiting beliefs, in order to expose the stories that we tell ourselves and come to terms with reality. 'The only time we suffer is when we believe a thought that argues with what is' (p.1).[1]

> A thought is harmless unless we believe it. It is not our thoughts, but the *attachment* to our thoughts, that causes suffering. Attaching to a thought means believing that it's true, without inquiring. A belief is a thought that we've been attaching to, often for years. (p.4, italics in the original)

It can be very interesting to reflect on why you are holding onto a particular limiting belief. Does it serve you in any way? Does it give you attention or get you out of doing something you don't want to do – or fulfil any other need? If you get everyone to believe that you're no good at washing up the dishes because you break stuff, you might get out of doing it every time. If you can recognize your limiting beliefs as a game you keep playing, it will be easier to take the decision to stop playing. There is still plenty of space to be compassionate towards yourself. It's okay that you had a limiting belief. It has served its purpose and now you are ready to discard it. Tell yourself, you are worthy of success, you can stand tall, you can take advantage of all the opportunities around you, and you can feel good about yourself.

PREJUDICES

Most of us are aware of and deal with our prejudices when they are the big, public issues where we need to be politically correct, such as age, sexuality, gender, socio-economic status, race or religion. But you also might have some smaller, personalized prejudices. For those who think they don't have any prejudices, see if you react to any of these:

- the parent who pacifies their two-year-old with sweets whenever they have a tantrum – and a couple of years later the child needs fillings in their milk teeth

---

1   Byron Katie's worksheets are available through her website, www.thework.com.

- the obese or anorexic teenager who comes to you for dietary advice but with every suggestion you make, they have a reason not to do it

- bicycle riders who jump the red light at traffic lights

- the dog lovers who allow their dogs to defecate on the pavement or near to the children's playpark

- people who play their music too loud.

If you don't agree that these are small, personal prejudices, then call them what you like. Perhaps they are personal values, community attitudes or socially accepted norms. Whatever you decide to call them, they are going to influence your perception of the patient as they hold a measure of prejudgement and intolerance. As a practitioner inquiring into a patient's symptoms, it is inevitable that on occasion you will uncover values or attitudes that are different from your own. Sometimes your reaction is lightweight and can easily be put aside, while at other times it needs a lot of self-reflection.

Prejudice can arise early on in the consultation if you recognize a similarity to a previous case, making you jump to conclusions about the disease diagnosis or treatment plan. Alternative practitioners are taught to treat each case as individual and requiring a personalized treatment plan. Choosing a prescription or treatment plan prior to understanding the whole story, amounts to prejudice. Samuel Hahnemann, the founder of homeopathy, advised practitioners to be the unprejudiced observer so that they understand each patient and their symptoms without prejudgement. Prescriptions are made on the individuality of the symptoms, not the disease diagnosis. Several patients might visit a homeopath with the same disease diagnosis, such as eczema. However, they will each be prescribed a different remedy according to the precise nature of each individual's symptoms including their moods and feelings. So it is important for the homeopath to listen carefully and observe the patient with accuracy.

Another way in which prejudice can arise very early on in the consultation is when you have expectations or prejudgements about the patient. Being neutral can be more difficult than it seems, because as soon as you meet your patient, you can unconsciously put them into a category or group according to your previous experience with similar people. This is not necessarily a prejudice or even a value judgement, but it can affect your expectations of the patient, the illness or the treatment outcome. A student who was being supervised by me admitted that he was deeply shocked when he was asked to treat an 82-year-old in clinic, and discovered that she wore a bright tracksuit and trainers and did yoga. His preconceptions were formed from his European childhood where women of grandmother age put on weight, moved slowly and wore black. The student found he could not relate easily to this dynamic, flexible, colourful and yet elderly lady.

The patient might say something that captures your attention because it resonates too much with you. Perhaps it reminds you of a similar experience in your own life; or perhaps it's an issue that has always pushed your buttons and irritated you. If this happens, your mind will start to chase after it, blocking out whatever the patient is currently talking about. It is surprising how rapidly the mind can switch from listening carefully to a patient – to an internal dialogue about a particular issue. It might even tempt you to consider self-disclosure to the patient, which in most cases is overstepping the ethical boundary.

There are times when patients surprise you or shock you because their values, opinions or attitudes are completely different to your own. Their behaviour might be outside of your experience. A mother who had three children under four placidly described how she would spend most of her time with the baby in the bedroom, leaving the other two to roam around the house. She would put a variety of sandwiches, crisps and quiche onto a small table, from which the three and four-year-old could graze all day. When her husband came in from work, he would hoover up the crumbs and cook an evening meal. I don't know which shocked me the most, the two little children having to fend for themselves or the calmness of the mother, recommending this as a system of child-rearing. She couldn't understand why other mothers made such a fuss about feeding their children. I was completely distracted from taking her case, and started to compare this behaviour to every other mother I had met, including myself. Within minutes I had made a moral judgement about her.

After she left I did some self-reflection and remembered how I had enjoyed listening to her for the first part of the consultation, as she was clever and witty. That memory helped remove some of my prejudice and I felt I could start analysing her case. Her indolence dated from the birth of the baby and repeated bouts of mastitis. It was more of a mental lethargy than a physical weakness. I considered her boasting about her system of child-rearing, which consisted of complacently going to bed with a good book and the baby. To this I added her physical symptoms of red, sore and cracked lips, mastitis with redness of nipples and dry skin that was aggravated when she had a shower. As I began to feel compassion for her, my prejudice fell away and I recognized which remedy I would like to prescribe. (The homeopathic remedy, *Sulphur*.)

Another form of prejudice arises from your inner self-talk which normally turns inwards, regularly commenting on your thoughts, emotions or activities and indulging in self-criticism or self-justification. However the same negative inner voice can be projected outwards onto a friend, a colleague or a patient. This is a form of transference or countertransference. One way to spot this happening is when your inner voice forgets to treat the other person as an individual, and starts to lay down laws about their behaviour. Even phrases like, 'They should' or 'They ought to' imply a standard that needs to be achieved. But who set that standard in the first place? Frequently it is voices from your own past rather than a universally held belief.

There are many different strategies that you can use to rid yourself of prejudices. It is very effective to talk them through with a supervisor, peer group or critical friend. Their questions will help you explore where the prejudice comes from and whether you have ever experienced the opposite of that prejudice.

A practitioner asked me for supervision because her patient had very different opinions and attitudes to hers. She felt she wanted to criticize her patient rather than feel empathy. Her patient came because of a problem with fibroids and heavy bleeding. She was in her early 50s and had a busy practice as a lawyer. She told the practitioner that she didn't regret not having children and that she was considerably irritated by small children. Sometimes when she went to the supermarket, her trolley would 'accidentally' hit young children walking in the aisles, and if she was in a hurry she would just push past them so that they fell over. She would just walk off, feeling justified, even if the child cried. The practitioner listening to this story was deeply shocked. She had children and grandchildren that she loved very much and her patient's behaviour seemed to her to be both violent and abusive.

As the supervisor, I wasn't going to advise the practitioner what to do with her patient, and I wasn't going to condone the patient's conduct. However, I was interested to see if I could get the practitioner to see the story from her patient's point of view – and having done that, whether she would feel a little compassion for the patient. She was not able to view the patient from the role of unprejudiced observer when she arrived and my aim was to get her more in that direction.

You can do the same exercise in your self-reflective journal. First write down what happened in your own words as you experienced it, without rewriting history. It might help to sit in your consulting room seat while you are doing this. Then, sitting in the patient's chair (or imagining you are) tell the same story from their point of view. This will become easier if you try sitting like them, speaking like them and making the same gestures. You have spent time focusing on this patient, and either consciously or unconsciously you know them very well.

Brian Kaplan (2001), writing in *The Homeopathic Conversation: The Art of Taking the Case*, recommends self-reflection:

> When I find myself judging a patient or unable to feel warmth towards him, I try to ask myself why this is so. The most frequent answer I get to this question is that up to the point of asking the question, I have unconsciously noticed in the patient a feature in myself that I dislike or am unable to accept. I then try to admit this to myself and accept myself as a whole in the moment. If I can accept the imperfection in myself, I can simultaneously accept it in the patient. (p.104)

Other ways of working with your prejudices in your journal, are to ask yourself such key reflective questions as: 'When/where have I felt like this before?' or 'What are my earliest memories of having this thought?'

A practitioner was asked if she would allow a guide dog into her clinic. She came to supervision because she had a strong dislike of animals. I asked what her first thought would be if she was on the bus and a teenager with a dog got on. She replied, 'They shouldn't allow dogs on buses.' She justified this with, 'Dogs are dirty.' These generalizations showed me that there were some un-thought-through judgements going on.

I asked her what her earliest memories of dogs were and she remembered her mother telling her never to go near dogs as they would bite her. She was very small at the time, and she had been obeying her mother's instructions ever since. I asked her whether there were any dogs that she liked and she described a couple of dogs on TV shows or movies. As we talked she began to realize that she had never really made the effort to get to know any real dog and maybe it was time to start.

Another way of working with your prejudice about a patient is to reflect on the positive, such as writing a list of ten things that you like about this patient or colleague (or dog). Focusing on the positive turns the limelight away from the aspects of this person that you are prejudiced about and makes you think positively about them. You can also make a list of the things you have in common with this person.

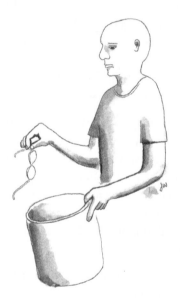

FIGURE 7.1: GET RID OF THOSE OLD GLASSES THAT DISTORT THE WORLD

ACCEPT WHAT IS

Having negative, preconceived ideas about yourself or about someone else is a bit like looking at the world through a constrictive mask or wearing glasses of the wrong prescription. You won't see clearly what is really going on (see Figure 7.1). The more you can be mindful, accepting of what is in this moment right now, the easier it will be to understand and heal your patient.

▰ REFLECTIVE EXAMPLE

A mother brought her four-year-old son to see me. She was well-dressed, drove a big car, her husband was a religious leader, and they had four children. Mother and son came to the consultation. When they arrived the boy (my patient) refused to enter the consulting room. His mother roughly pushed him in, and once he was in he went to the toys, with his back to us. There was no other contact between them. I explained to him about the case-taking, but he ignored me, and the mother just smiled, so I directed the case-taking to her.

Her manner was calm, her smile was bland and rather emotionless, and her voice level. She told me a lot of unpleasant things about her son, his rude and stubborn behaviour, his poor toileting, his lack of learning, and so on. I felt uncomfortable that the son was hearing all of this.

He continued to play, and did not react to anything she said. Finally, I felt I wanted to include him some more, and asked him directly about his food desires. He turned to me and made several rude and unpleasant noises and gestures, and then returned to his toys. His mother took no notice, and smiled at me blandly again, while answering the question herself.

What were my thoughts and feelings?

At the time, my feelings were of awkwardness, and embarrassment. When he was so rude to me, I suppose I was expecting the mother to gently admonish him, or show me an expression of apology, but her acceptance of his behaviour surprised and embarrassed me.

After the consultation, I found myself thinking more and more about the strange relationship between these two, rather like irritable next-door neighbours rather than mother and child. The mother's interest was detached, as if this was not her blood relation. The child just demanded negative attention. I found myself wondering how she treated her other children, and why she had four children if she did not enjoy their company. I was unable to let go of this situation.

What concerns me about this case?

- Usually I can make children relax, or the mother helps me to relate to them. In this case, I felt that she was colluding with his rude behaviour, although she was probably just demonstrating how she usually ignores him.

- I was surprised by the situation of a dysfunctional family masquerading as a close knit, happy, religious leader's family. They would be on show to all of the community.

Discussion

The first issue for me is that both the mother and child have been rude to me, the child directly and the mother indirectly by not apologizing for his behaviour. I felt shocked and surprised, because I had been doing my best to help this family.

I think I am assuming that all patients come to me voluntarily and want to have their case taken. But this is not true when the patient is a child. This child made it very clear he did not want to enter the clinic room or take part in the consultation. Perhaps he had heard his mother list all of his faults too many times before. His rudeness was towards his mother as well as me.

The mother is more difficult to analyse. She chose to make the appointment for her son, but she took no responsibility for his behaviour. There is a coldness about her that has triggered my prejudices. My inner critical voice says she is masquerading as a loving mother and religious leader's wife, as if she ought to do better. I need to unpack this. The reality is that she is not masquerading at all. It is my imagination, my delusion that she ought to be an example for the rest of the community and that she pretends to be a more loving parent in front of them. But from what I have seen, she is indifferent or unable to express any love. I'm beginning to question whether she is very depressed or whether she is on some sort of medication. There is a lot more going on in this family than I have been told or understood.

Thinking about her being depressed makes me more compassionate towards her. She has had several children close together.

Action possibilities

- If the mother returns with the child for a follow-up, then I need to be prepared. I will do my favourite protection ritual before they come, and spend a few minutes in mindful meditation.

- I could ask if the boy's behaviour is typical. I'm interested to know if he's like this with other people.

- I could ask the mother how she feels about his behaviour. She does not mind talking about painful things in front of the son.

- It would be interesting to ask the mother how she felt about the pregnancy. I'm curious to know whether she has always felt negatively towards this son and if so, how he reacted to her.

- I could suggest to the mother that she comes for treatment as well.

- If they are rude to me again, or another patient is rude, I should do some clearing exercises after the consultation, so that I do not hold onto my hurt feelings.

- I can take it to my supervisor to discuss further. Maybe I have other layers of prejudice that I haven't spotted yet.

EXERCISE: EXPLORING YOUR LIMITING BELIEFS

Ask yourself what it is that you regularly say that you are no good at. Writing in your reflective journal, ask why, like a curious child. Ask why 10 or 20 times, each time going to a deeper level. If you come to a halt because you have found the ideal excuse such as blaming someone else, then pause and then start again. For example:

I'm no good at maths.

Why? I found it difficult at school.

Why? Because I didn't bother to study it.

Why? Because my friends and I thought it was boring.

Why? Because we couldn't see any practical use in it.

Why? Because the teacher didn't relate it to the real world.

Pause: I want to blame the teacher.

Why? Because that's easier than looking to myself.

Why?

EXERCISE: EXPLORING YOUR LIMITING BELIEFS

Choose one of your limiting beliefs, something that you think that you are no good at. Then assuming the role of the unprejudiced observer, ask yourself, *Is it true? Is it really true?* Write a list in your journal of all the times that you have been effective in some small way in the subject that you denigrate yourself for. Make a list of all the small things that you manage to do effectively within the scope of your limiting belief. When you have finished, ask yourself again if you're really so deficient in that skill or experience. Then ask yourself why you need to put yourself down about it.

EXERCISE: UNCOVERING YOUR PREJUDICES

Choose a picture from magazines or the Internet of the type of patient that you do not want to come into your consulting room. Show the picture to a critical friend who will ask you why you do not want this patient coming to see you. The critical friend should repeatedly ask why, to reveal the different layers of truth.

EXERCISE: UNCOVERING YOUR PREJUDICES

Identify one thing that you are prejudiced about when it comes to other people, something that your critical inner voice freely denounces, like they are too thin, too fat, speak too fast, move too slow, don't say enough, talk too much, too self-pitying, too concerned with other people, has too much fun or takes life too seriously. Take a blank sheet of paper and fold it in half. Draw a picture of this person on half of the page, and then folding the paper so that the first drawing is out of sight, draw yourself on the other half of the page. Finally open up the paper so that you can see both drawings side-by-side. What can you learn from this?

EXERCISE: SELF-COMPASSION

Reflect on your achievements in the past, however small and then write two lists. The first list is of things that you expected to achieve. Begin the other list with the words, 'I never thought I would...' With the implication that you're pleased you did achieve in that area after all.

In the first list you could write: I expected to get at least four GCSEs and I got six, I expected to leave home at 18 and I did. In the second list write the things that surprised you: I never thought I would get over my fear of dogs, I never thought I would graduate from my acupuncture course, I never thought I would pass my driving test, I never thought I would learn how to bake cakes – but I did!

The second list has the things that you should be really proud of. There was some sort of limiting belief holding you back, and yet you still achieved mastery. Take your time with this; don't toss it aside as a second-class achievement. You succeeded in it despite being held back by a limiting belief, and this marks it as a major achievement. It was tough for you, and you had to work at your own pace, but you got there in the end. Your success was all the more welcome because of the difficult journey to get there. You have done it once and you can do it again!

Chapter 8

PLANNING THE WAY FORWARD

After the practitioner has taken the case and fully understands all they need to make a prescription or decide on a treatment, the consultation moves on to the next phase. This is the negotiation and planning stage. It may only take five minutes, but it is crucial to the on-going relationship between practitioner and patient. It can happen partway through the session, when the practitioner stops interviewing and is ready to do a treatment, or it can happen at the end of the session.

In a medical setting, this would be the point when the doctor makes a diagnosis and explains it to the patient, giving the official name of the disease, showing how the symptoms are related to this and making a prescription or a recommendation for further tests. Alternative practitioners very rarely name diseases in this way. Many alternative therapies are supported by complex Eastern philosophies that see a disease as a result of underlying imbalance. For most of us the primary aim is to get the system back into balance again, whereupon the disease would no longer have the conditions in which to thrive. Homeopathy has its origins in Germany, but has a similar philosophy of treating the underlying imbalance first.

Although alternative practitioners don't give a diagnosis as such, the patient still deserves to hear what your conclusions are and what you recommend. The temptation might be to give this in terms of your underlying philosophy, but for most patients that is as helpful as a doctor speaking Latin. You will need a simplified explanation of the theory to give to patients, and you might have to memorize a few key sentences that they can understand. If they want to know more than this, they will ask. You can explain what treatment you recommend, your prognosis about how healing will progress, whether there will be any treatment reaction and how many appointments they may need.

The patient might not be very receptive to being given large amounts of information at this stage. They might be feeling tired or emotional after talking or sleepy after a treatment; or they might be feeling vulnerable and not want to think about the next step. There are a few things that you can do to help them. You can use short, clear, understandable sentences and keep away from jargon. Silverman *et al.* (2005) write:

> If you give information in small chunks and give the patient ample opportunity to contribute, they will respond with clear signals about both the amount and type of information they still require. (p.158)

FEEDBACK AND PROGNOSIS

If you have a few different things that you're going to recommend, you can use the technique of signposting. This means saying what you're going to say before you say it. It is a brief summary of each issue that you're hoping to cover, like the list of contents at the front of the book, so that people know what to expect. Then you explain each point in turn. Sometimes a prepared handout will help them remember. Visual aids, even just a quick drawing, help many people to understand what you're saying, especially if they can take a copy home as a visual reminder.

With some disciplines, the practitioner does not reach their conclusion within the consultation time. In these cases you should explain why there will be a delay, and when they can expect your feedback and recommendations.

Having given your prognosis on the patient's condition, told them how many treatments or prescriptions might be necessary and whether any treatment reaction is likely, you should now turn to the patient and ask how that suits them. Where possible, you should offer them choices about aspects of the treatment. You should involve them in the decision-making process and negotiate the overall treatment plan.

As a homeopath, I felt there were two areas which I could negotiate with the patient, and one area that only I could decide. I was the only one who could choose the remedy because of my training and my many years of experience. But I could ask the patient which potency (strength) of the remedy they would prefer. I might offer a single dose in tablet form which would give them a speedy result, but which might cause an aggravation of the presenting symptoms or an emotional outburst. The alternative could be a lower potency with less aggravation, or a liquid dose taken on a daily basis. The patient could also choose when they wanted the next appointment.

Once you have negotiated and reached a joint treatment plan, ask them if they have any questions or if there is anything they want further clarification on. With some patients, you might want to reiterate the treatment plan just before they leave and with many you will need to put it in writing. In most cases the treatment plan becomes part of the working agreement.

The TV series *House* is a sitcom about a bad-tempered, controlling and very rude doctor in a hospital, played by Hugh Laurie. His patient for one episode is a woman returning to the clinic to say that her inhaler didn't help her asthma. He asks if she understands how to use it properly, and she indignantly replies, of course. He then asks her to demonstrate and she sprays the inhaler behind her ears as if it was perfume. Dr House can hardly prevent himself from laughing in her face. This is an exaggerated scenario and extremely funny, but it does highlight how there can be a complete mismatch between what the practitioner prescribes and what the patient understands.

Occasionally, the patient does not want to think about their treatment plan. They might be elderly and used to a Parent–Child practitioner–patient relationship. Or they may be too tired or anxious to make rational choices, and just want to hand over the decision-making to the practitioner. This is fine if they want to follow your recommendations, but the danger is that you will be put on a pedestal as the 'expert' and made to hold all of the responsibility. I suggest that you still continue to explain everything and make sure the patient understands what you are offering, and agrees with the plan.

ASKING THE PATIENT TO DO HOMEWORK

All health practitioners want the best for their patients mentally, emotionally and physically. According to your therapy, you will be expecting the patient to share the responsibility for the improvement in their health to a greater or lesser extent. Some therapies rely solely on the work done within the treatment session, but many involve the patient doing a positive activity at home, such as changing the diet, practising certain exercises, taking prescriptions or getting to bed earlier.

Referring back to the three ego states model (see Chapter 3), as a practitioner your choice is either to take a Parental role and treat the patient as a Child, or to communicate on an Adult–Adult level. If you choose the former, you will be taking the role of the expert who knows best and who demands compliance from the patient. This is the old doctor–patient model from 50 or 100 years ago and it puts all of the responsibility into the hands of the doctor.

As you probably know from your own experience as a patient, this attitude can create resistance, non-compliance or non-return of the patient. On the other hand, if you choose the Adult role, you invite them to go into their Adult role, from where you can involve them in the treatment plan. This means inviting them to comment on your suggestions and contribute their ideas and thoughts as to how they can help improve their health. In return you will be getting a good idea of how realistic your recommendations are and you can revise them accordingly.

BOX 8.1 NEGOTIATING FOR CHANGE

- Make your suggestions clear
- Use simple language with no jargon
- Use visual aids and printed handouts
- Check the patient's understanding
- Observe the patient's body language
- Use listening skills when the patient speaks
- Compromise if necessary
- Collaborate on an Adult–Adult level

Try to explain your recommendations as carefully as possible, using simple language and handouts or visual aids. Listen to the patient's point of view with courtesy and respect – and watch their body language carefully. If it becomes apparent that what you're asking is too difficult for the patient, consider a compromise. Maybe they are just not ready to follow your recommendations. Perhaps your suggestions were too complex or far-reaching and you need to make it simpler and more manageable for them. Maybe they can come up with better suggestions.

Sharing the responsibility with the patient has several ramifications. When you invite them to contribute their thoughts and feelings about a treatment plan, you empower them. Their suggestions about how they can contribute can be excellent. Involving the patient in their own treatment plan reduces the burden on you so that you become more of a facilitator rather than an expert. But for some patients sharing the responsibility can be frightening or overwhelming. It means they would have to take responsibility for actively improving their health in certain areas that they have not wanted to think about for many years. Old habits, however destructive they are of health and self, have the appeal of the familiar.

At times I have set this up as a role-play for my students. The 'practitioner' had to persuade the 'patient' to make some lifestyle changes, such as stopping smoking, losing weight, or getting more exercise. The students were asked to think about this beforehand and make notes about what they wanted to say. Those in practitioner role wrote out lists of why the current behaviour was bad for the patient and what they could do to improve their lifestyle. Their arguments ranged from medical research to the good feeling factor. Meanwhile the patients were preparing emotional or stubborn counterarguments, such as their addiction to cigarettes or overeating was necessary as a de-stressor, or that they simply didn't feel ready to change. You can imagine the gridlock that ensued.

Following this role-play, I ask the students to discuss in small groups other ways of approaching the issue of lifestyle change with their patients. I then ask them to give concrete examples of how they would negotiate. Here are some of the suggestions they came up with:

- Ask the patient what medical research they have read or heard of with regards to the health issue that you want them to change.

- Ask them if they have any suggestions about what they can do to help themselves.

- Explain that shared responsibility and teamwork between practitioner and patient are often the most effective way to achieve results.

- Give them any new information so that they can make an informed choice.

- Don't let the patient take on too much at once.

- Start with something small and realistic that the patient can achieve and feel good about, and build up from there as the patient progresses.

- Make all suggestions and instructions in the positive (what they should do) and not in the negative (what they shouldn't do).

- Decide how often the patient should check in with the practitioner to report back (and receive praise).

- Design a soft reward system that does not include anything illegal, immoral or fattening, such as buying a new book to read, visiting a friend or going to the beach.

- Write down the joint decision in the patient's notes and offer a printed version for them to keep.

- Have some 'what if?' strategies prepared.

- Be compassionate! We have all broken resolutions at times, but a few days of forgetting can always be followed by getting back into the routine again.

Some of these are self-evident, but some need further explanation. Making all suggestions in the positive is an interesting point. We always tell our children, 'Don't do this', 'Don't touch', 'Don't forget', using the negative form of the instruction. But many children, especially the young ones, cannot hear the negative. Their brains understand the instruction as, 'Do this', 'Touch' and 'Forget'. It would be much clearer to them if adults could say, 'Keep away' and 'Remember'. Small children are right-brain dominant, and the patient who has just recalled their story or who has just received a treatment is in a temporary right-brain state. Neighbour (2005) writes about the two sides of the brain:

> The right hemisphere doesn't understand negation. It responds to negatives as if they weren't there. To the right hemisphere: **don't** means **do**, **won't** means **might**, **can't** means **could**, and **shouldn't** means **probably will**. (p.186, emphasis in the original)

If the patient has been told to check in regularly with the practitioner, they need plenty of praise for what they have achieved rather than comments about what they haven't. Criticism will not motivate them to work harder towards their goal. It is more likely to make them give up entirely.

The patient should be given a written copy of the negotiated treatment plan, because the consultation is set up so that the patient is in explaining mode for most of the time. They are thinking about their condition and telling their story, and many are not ready for the turnaround of having to receive information towards the end of the session. It is as if they are too full of their own words to hear the words of the practitioner. Some of you might have experienced this, walking out of the doctor's surgery with absolutely no recall of what the doctor has just told you, even though you nodded and smiled and said you understood at the time.

Some people have held onto their bad habits for a long time and maybe they need to wean themselves of it very slowly, such as a smoker reducing their number of cigarettes every week. You might have to say to the patient, 'We might not achieve your goal within these conditions/this time frame, but we can certainly start you off in the right direction.'

With some patients and some conditions, it is useful to have some 'what if' strategies prepared in advance. A situation where this might occur is when someone has recurring acute pain, and both of you have decided you would like to reduce the amount of painkillers that are taken. These might be headaches, period pains or aching joints; all cases where you have explained that they will need several appointments before it will be cured. The question that arises is: what if they get another acute bout in the meantime? The strategies might include going for a walk, taking a warm shower, drinking plenty of plain water, cutting out stimulants, doing a three-minute meditation, distracting themselves by dancing to their favourite music or taking a nap for an hour.

Compassion is a key ingredient during negotiations for change. Your inner voice might want to say, 'If you really want to lose weight or stop smoking, just do it!' Technically, you would be right, the patient is the only person who can lose their weight or stop their smoking. Take a moment to remember the time when you found yourself stuck and unable to do something that you knew was obvious and sensible – but the safety and familiarity of the old habits kept you from moving forwards. We have all been there and need to remember our experiences in common with the patient. You will be a much more effective motivator if you can come from a place of compassion rather than criticism.

PREPARED HANDOUTS

Over the years I made up several help-yourself handouts for my patients on such diverse topics as children's fevers, cystitis, or menopause. These are empowering because they have suggestions of different self-help measures my patients could do at home. All of my handouts state clearly that if the condition becomes worse, they should contact their doctor or alternative practitioner. The self-help measures mainly comprise of old 'folk' remedies and wise woman suggestions, such as changing the diet or changing the clothes.

For example, my handout on stomach upsets includes pointers on loose clothing, personal hygiene, stopping stimulants, making your own rehydration fluid and the BRAT diet. BRAT refers to bananas, rice, apples (grated raw apple or apple sauce) and toast, and can be suggested for patients with diarrhoea or gastroenteritis. Variations are BRATT which includes tea; and BRATTY which includes tea and yoghurt.

Other handouts could be visual aids such as simple drawings of exercises that you recommend or pulse points that you want the patient to massage during an acute episode.

COLLABORATION

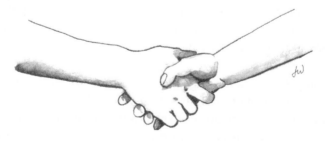

FIGURE 8.1: REACH A COOPERATIVE AGREEMENT

In the last century there was a lot of concern about patient compliance: patients were not doing what they were told. In this century there has been a movement towards negotiating a joint treatment plan. This doesn't suit everyone, but generally patients are better informed and more interested in taking part in their own healing. A cooperative agreement is often more realistic than a fixed prescription, and being encouraged to do something for themselves between appointments, can be very empowering for the patient. The practitioner saves time and is relieved from the frustration of the patient returning, saying they are no better but confessing to have not followed instructions. Beyond this, collaboration creates a feel-good factor for both people.

REFLECTIVE EXAMPLE

A man came to see me at the clinic for a treatment. I have to admit I've never met anyone like him before, and I was puzzled. He seemed very impatient, and was very abrupt with me when I tried to tell him about the treatment agreement, saying, 'Yes, yes, I'm sure it's all on your website.' He relaxed during the treatment but afterwards, when I tried to plan for the future with him, he became abrupt again. He said he didn't want to book another appointment until he could see how this treatment affected him. I tried to explain that his problem was long-term but he got stuck with the idea that he should feel incrementally better after each individual treatment. We were on completely different wavelengths and rather than argue with him, I gave up. I will know that if he books in again, it will be because he felt better this evening. In the meantime I have decided to 'step into his shoes' as an experiment in my journal, to see what I can learn.

(Later) what an interesting experiment! I sat quietly for a while just trying to reconnect with what he was like, and then mimed him coming into the clinic. He walked fast, with a mixture of rushing and then hesitating, so he was in the centre of the room before I could close the door, but then he hesitated because he didn't know where to sit. Then I mimed him sitting on the chair as I went through my questions. He was quite restless moving around in his chair, and when I stopped to check my textbook, he checked his texts on his phone. I tried moving as much as he did and I began to feel impatient and fidgety. He looked around my clinic room quite a lot, and when I did that, I felt myself losing concentration.

When I mimed him, I felt as if I had little time and a lot of work to do. I felt like someone who has been living a stressful life for a long time, feeling permanently rushed, always having something else to do — and (this last one just popped into my head!) being surrounded by incompetent people. I wonder if that is what he really felt like? Am I just guessing? Let me think this through. If his experience is that he is rushed, has no time, feels impatient, feels overworked and feels other people are incompetent, then my session with its opening discussion must have felt very slow for him. I can imagine him questioning my competency, because he probably does that with most people. I can imagine him letting go completely and relaxing during the session, but as soon as it was over he went back into stress mode again. He would need more treatments (at least six, probably ten) so that his body can learn how to relax again when he is at home. The question is: will he be patient enough to come back for more treatments?

Aha! Even if this is just guessing, it is very useful to consider what might have been his motivations. I understand him much better now, and feel more trust that he will return. His rather abrasive manner won't upset me so much a second time round, and he will remember how well he relaxed during the first treatment. To help him, I can speak clearly and to the point.

EXERCISE: NEGOTIATING YOUR HOMEWORK

Imagine you have decided to go to a new practitioner (therapy of your choice) and you're coming to the end of your consultation with them. You have got on well with them and told them a lot about your life. You have had the opportunity to ask some questions, and you are interested to see what they prescribe or what treatment plan they suggest. To your surprise they pick out two of your bad habits and tell you that they would like you to begin improving these before your next appointment. Consider which two bad habits would you find particularly difficult to change? They might be around your diet, caffeine intake, lack of exercise, negative thinking, forgetfulness in one key area, obsessive behaviour or sleep routines. How easily will you take to changing these when your practitioner asks you?

EXERCISE: MOTIVATING YOUR PATIENT

Consider what inducements you can use to get your patient to change their habits. Start with thinking about your manner; what sort of body language would motivate them? Does it need confidence, enthusiasm, friendliness, compassion, interest, forcefulness or anything else? Think about the words you would use and your tone of voice. How can you point out unhelpful behaviour in a way that is supportive? Help them to phrase a motivating mantra for themselves, or compile a list of soft rewards they can give themselves.

Chapter 9

SETTING AND MAINTAINING BOUNDARIES

Relationship boundaries are the personal guidelines or limits we create in our behaviour towards others and our expectation of other's behaviour towards us; and how we respond if someone oversteps those guidelines. For many people, having personal codes of reasonable, permissible behaviour gives them security and self-respect. They know what feels right in their attitude towards others and others to them. Boundaries are a protection device, clarifying the difference between *me* and *not-me*.

Professional boundaries are a refined version of these guidelines which are appropriate and effective for interaction between practitioner and patient. They are written into the code of conduct or code of ethics for each therapy, but in an umbrella format that does not give detailed strategies. Each practitioner has to make their own decisions about where they want to set their boundaries.

When a practitioner and patient work together, the boundary lines become more complex than with a personal relationship. The patient is vulnerable, while the practitioner is knowledgeable. Does this mean the practitioner should relax their personal boundaries and do more for the patient, or does it mean the practitioner should increase their boundaries and thereby control the patient? How much should the patient be treated as vulnerable and needing compassion, and how much should the patient be viewed with caution because they are manipulative?

Many people don't know where their boundaries are set, until they are challenged. If you feel discomfort or worse still, indignation after a consultation or patient communication, this is probably a warning signal that your boundaries have been transgressed. Su Fox writes that you can learn to recognize your somatic responses when someone intrudes into your personal space, such as tight jaw, clenched hands, shallow breathing, holding the breath, tight shoulder muscles and so on (2008, pp.64–65). These may be accompanied by negative thoughts, such as the patient is taking liberties or demanding too much.

On realizing that your boundaries have been pushed, you need to reflect on why this has happened and what needs to be done. It might mean that you have to re-contract either with this patient or across the whole practice. There is no problem with this as long as you are open and transparent about it. You don't need to explain your reasons for re-contracting, just state clearly what is in the new contract. For instance, you might find that telling a patient to phone if there is a problem was misunderstood as, 'Phone any time day or night.' Your new, refreshed contract would have to include something like, 'Phone calls are answered between 9am and 5pm.'

BOUNDARIES CREATE STRUCTURE

The advantage of boundaries are that they create a firm structure or framework within which you and your patient can interact with flexibility and safety. They provide a guideline to acceptable behaviour that protects and respects both you and your patients. For example, having time boundaries means that both of you know when the consultation will start and when it will end. Without clear time boundaries you would have to sit in the clinic all day waiting for the patient to turn up.

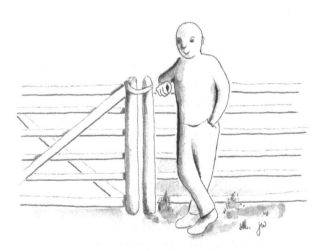

FIGURE 9.1: PROTECT YOURSELF WITH A CLEAR BOUNDARY.
YOU CAN CHOOSE WHEN TO OPEN THE GATE

You need to create boundaries and keep them in place in order to set up a safe and supportive environment for everyone. But having set these up for the whole of the practice, you should still be able to loosen your boundaries for particular patients or circumstances (see Figure 9.1). There are times when either your carefully considered logic or your intuition tells you that the blurring of *this* boundary for *that* patient is appropriate. For example, a practitioner who clearly states in all of their literature they don't do home visits, might choose to visit their long-term patient at home while they have a broken leg. Without a certain amount of flexibility there would be no room for compassion. Santorelli (1999) reminds us that boundaries can be variable:

> The usual meaning of boundary is 'dividing line' – a separation between two things. But isn't a boundary also a place of meeting and coming together? When walking barefoot along the shoreline, are we only on the land? What about the water under our feet? Where does the land begin and end? Where exactly is the water's edge? (p.61)

On the other hand, if boundaries are always unclear or constantly changing, the shoreline can become quicksand, leading to a confused patient at best – and a complicated, dysfunctional or unprofessional relationship at worst. The patient who gets confused or embarrassed by unclear boundaries is often the one that does not return.

Newly qualified homeopaths can get very confused about money boundaries. It's a problem that doesn't happen with hands-on therapies and has been made worse with the invention of electronic communication. Should they charge for every phone or text query from established patients? What about phone consultations? How much should they charge for a Skype appointment? When should they ask the patient to come in and pay for an appointment? As a result charges can be quite variable which makes the practitioner feel awkward and puzzles the patient. The answer is to quite ruthlessly calculate the fees for everything and write them down. This gives the practitioner a baseline to work from and if they want to charge less they can say to the patient, 'I normally charge this amount, but for this call I will only charge so much/I won't be charging.' Then the patient knows where they stand.

Money is necessary as part of the transaction between practitioner and patient in the private sector, but the boundaries need to be set very early on. You cannot suddenly surprise the patient by telling them they need to pay more than the advertised price.

PHYSICAL BOUNDARIES

One way of looking at physical boundaries is to consider the senses of sight, hearing, smell and touch. You probably want your clinic room to look reasonably professional and business-like without being cold or stark. If you're using a room within your house or apartment, you need to decide how much of your private life is revealed, and to what extent the clinic room is made to look professional and impersonal. If the room appears too much like the family sitting room, or the consultation is around the kitchen table, the patient will receive the unspoken message that they can be friendly and casual. This can have the knock-on effect of poor timekeeping, erratic fee-paying, and generally not taking your work seriously.

Your clinic room should be reasonably soundproof so that when the door is closed the patient can speak in confidence without worrying that their consultation might be overheard by others. Phones can be set on a silent mode, and in most cases should not be answered during a patient consultation.

I was once sent to a doctor in a busy hospital. The previous patient came out of the room, but I was left waiting in the corridor for 20 or 30 minutes. When the doctor finally called me in, she explained that she was having computer problems, and that she'd been trying to phone the IT technicians but they hadn't answered her phone call yet. This was why she had kept me waiting. Feeling a sense of urgency about her computer, and unwilling to lose her place in the queue, she left the phone on loudspeaker. We conducted the consultation to the call-waiting music, punctuated by an optimistic recorded voice telling us that they knew we were waiting, and that our call was important to them. I was highly amused at a time, but as I left and wished the doctor good luck with her computer, I realized that the relationship had changed and I was no longer taking her seriously.

The windows of your clinic are there to let in light, but for confidentiality they can be shaded from people looking in. As far as possible, you can avoid strong smells in the room although some are unavoidable, such as using massage oils or burning moxa – or the previous patient's perfume or aftershave.

If you have to make a home visit, for whatever reason, a bedroom or sitting room may be used as a temporary clinic. This can make it challenging for you to uphold the normal protocols and boundaries of the session and it might be more difficult to maintain confidentiality. Your concentration can be broken by the distractions of phones, music, TV or other people in the building. If you make yourself 'at home' in a patient's home, the practitioner–patient relationship is challenged. The patient might want to show you their appreciation for a home visit by offering cups of tea or showing photos, but it is time spent as a guest rather than as a visiting practitioner.

PERSONAL SPACE

Physical boundaries also include the distance between the two people in the consulting room: the personal space. What defines a comfortable distance can vary between different races, cultures or societies, and the practitioner is left to decide what feels good. Su Fox (2008) reminds us that a personal space boundary:

> Is not a fixed space but one that expands or contracts depending on our environment, who we are with, our health and how tired we are. It is also partly determined by the culture that we grew up in. (p.63)

She goes on to say that even if the patient has agreed for a body-worker to enter their personal space, we should not take it for granted that the patient feels relaxed about it. The patient should be allowed to say if a particular area feels uncomfortable when approached or touched. I learned this lesson through an experience in which I was quite simply thoughtless. I had come to the end of the consultation with a patient and she was about to leave, when she suddenly went into a stomach cramp and bent over in pain. Visually this triggered memories in me of a friend who had similar cramps, and I automatically put my arm around her, with my palm against the cramp. She started up in horror, saying, 'What are you doing, what are you doing?' I dropped my arm immediately and apologized for the inappropriate touch. I should have asked her what she needed.

In the talking therapies, such as counselling or homeopathy, too much eye contact can be felt as an invasion of personal space. You should take this into account if the room is small or over-furnished so that the chairs feel forced up against each other. You could make the space more comfortable by offsetting the chairs or placing a small foliage plant between the two people. In a very large room where the open space feels intimidating, you can place the chairs or treatment couch so that only a small proportion of the room is visible.

If the patient needs to undress for acupuncture or body-work, you need to consider how the patient can undress with dignity, such as behind a screen or being left alone for a few minutes in the clinic room. Physical examinations for diagnosis should only be done if the practitioner has had appropriate training.

EMOTIONAL BOUNDARIES

Physical and spatial boundaries are quite easy to assess and maintain, compared to emotional boundaries. How much should the practitioner become involved in the patient's story? To fully understand the patient you need to feel empathy or compassion, and this means a commitment to feeling as well as hearing the patient's story. It is not enough to just hear the facts like a recording device. The patient only gives their story to someone who is empathizing and sharing this through facial expressions and body language. Entering the patient's world is the only way to understand them and help them, but risks your involvement. Babette Rothschild (2006) explains:

> Empathy is a multifaceted evolutionary phenomenon that facilitates the binding of people to each other. Knowing what another is feeling or feeling the same emotion oneself is a result of empathy. This ability has played a major role in the development of humankind by making it possible for individuals to bond into couples and groups, and to care for and socialize their young. (p.34)

When you are in close contact with other people, as in a relationship or in a consultation, you will spontaneously and unconsciously copy each other's facial expressions and body language. Families copy one another and develop the same mannerisms, including the family dog!

A stranger who smiles directly at you will usually raise a corresponding smile on your face. You experience the same reaction when you are watching a movie, and your body responds in parallel with the actor, so that when they weep, laugh or shrug their shoulders you feel yourself reacting in the same way. These often go unnoticed because they can be minute. It is probably the same process going on when you find yourself copying someone else's accent or turn of phrase, while you are talking to them. When interviewing a patient you will copy their facial expressions, gestures and body language. Once a patient unconsciously perceives you are mirroring them, they recognize that you are showing empathy and they open up and trust you with their story.

The downside of empathy is that it is always going on. Your brain automatically receives information from any other person that you focus on and converts it into a physical feeling or emotion, thus allowing you to feel what they feel. This is the action of the mirror neurons in the brain that copy or mirror other people, and it can be particularly intense during a consultation (see Chapter 12's section 'Separating from the patient').

If a lot of time is spent mirroring negative emotions conveyed by body language and facial expression, your brain cells can misinterpret this as an authentic emotion belonging to you. If you are unaware of this process, you might experience your patient's emotions or sensations and wonder where they come from. By the time you get home, you can find yourself unreasonably emotional – unreasonable in the sense that you cannot find a reason for it – because your anger, depression or sadness has come from your patient.

This is sometimes called emotional contagion as the emotions spread this way from one person to another like an infectious disease. A few small changes to your body language and eye contact can reduce this possibility. At your most empathetic you will probably be giving a lot of eye contact, with your own eyes wide open and soft, and your body language will be mirroring that of the other person. Try to consciously break the eye contact on a regular basis, even only to glance away for a few seconds. Deliberately change your body language every so often so that you don't continuously mirror their position or gestures.

Another way you can guard against absorbing the patient's emotions, is to set up a brief protection ritual that is done before the consultation. You can imagine yourself inside a protective bubble, or draw three circles in the air around them, front to back, side to side and horizontally around the waist (see Chapter 12's section 'Separating from the patient' for more ideas).

Getting to know yourself through supervision and self-reflection will increase your ability to observe the patient's emotional state and not feel overwhelmed by it. It will increase your compassion without attaching you to the patient's story. For instance, the patient might feel the need to express strong emotion during the consultation or the treatment, such as weeping or expressing anger. If you do not know yourself and understand your own reactions, you might feel the need to comfort the weeping patient or contain the anger of the irritated patient. Before giving in to your own impulses, you should check in with yourself who would benefit from this. It might have the effect of drying up the patient's tears or anger and preventing them from experiencing the emotion as a healthy discharge.

The other amazing tool for effectively being with the patient during the consultation and detaching from them afterwards, is mindfulness (see Chapter 5). Mindfulness means being in the present moment, just accepting what is, with loving warmth but without judgement and without looking forward to the future or back into the past. The effect this has on you is to stop your brain multitasking, which makes you more accepting of whatever comes up in the consultation.

One of the situations where it could become difficult to maintain emotional boundaries, is when the patient has a mental illness. This can make them suspicious of you or the opposite, wanting to be more intimate. To protect both of you, I suggest starting with a very strong working agreement with them that states clearly your availability, how long each session will last, how and when you can be contacted out of hours, your fees and so on. Make sure that the parent, carer or doctor is informed of their treatment plan with you.

DUAL RELATIONSHIPS

If you practise in a small community, the likelihood of dual relationships increases. Dual relationships are when practitioner and patient meet under different circumstances as well as in the clinic. It could be that you are neighbours or acquaintances, you have the same hobby, the patient is in a different service industry and has helped you in that role, one of you is teacher and the other is student, or you have two different skills and see the patient in both capacities. All of these can lead to a confusion of the working agreement and an overlapping of boundaries. Information from one relationship can get carried over to the other one, which can be detrimental to the healing process.

In a larger community, the ethical advice is to refer the patient on to another practitioner so they do not have to experience a dual relationship. In a small community where dual relationships cannot be avoided, you have to work extra hard to keep the boundaries in place. Your aim should be to keep each relationship 'clean' without seepage from the others. You should discuss this with the patient when you first set up the working agreement, so that you both keep the two relationships compartmentalized.

I recommend that you don't even consider treating friends or relatives. You know too much about them and cannot be in the role of unprejudiced observer. Or you might think you know all about them, when it was only one facet that you know so well.

A practitioner came to me for supervision as she wanted to talk about a patient, who was pushing her boundaries and upsetting her. This patient used to be a good friend of hers and had become one of her student cases. These student cases were taken in her apartment, and afterwards they would have a chat over a cup of tea. The arrangement worked really well, and the student practitioner did not charge fees to her friend. After graduation the practitioner explained to her friend that she would have to start charging fees, as she needed to pay for a clinic room. The friend agreed, but still wanted to spend time chatting at the end of each consultation; and if the practitioner did not have another appointment booked, the friend would suggest they went out for tea. The practitioner couldn't see how she could make stronger boundaries with the friend who had been so loyal to her during her training.

I sympathized with her because I could see how she was pulled in both directions between the old friend and the desire to be professional in her practice. I started off by getting her to think about dual relationships. This was a new idea to her, but she could reflect on it and realized how much she had learned from the experience. Then we had a brainstorming session to consider all the different actions she could take with her friend. She decided that she valued the old friendship above having another patient on her books.

The next time I saw her she told me that she had explained to her friend the difficulty with dual relationships, she had recommended a couple of local practitioners for her to try out, the friend had stopped being a patient – and they had been on a really fun girls' night out.

SEXUAL BOUNDARIES

If a practitioner has a brisk practice, and sees many different patients over the years, it seems to me to be inevitable that sooner or later they will find someone that, in another lifetime, they would have liked as a new friend or a sexual partner. But if you are a practitioner they have come to consult, these sorts of relationships are totally unethical.

As soon as you become aware of any sexual feelings, you need to do some self-reflection and ask yourself: can you contain your feelings, or should you stop seeing the patient? These are the only two options available, as practitioners should always fulfil their emotional and sexual needs outside of the working environment. Within the clinic and outside of it, it is your responsibility to ensure that neither you nor the patient crosses emotional or sexual boundaries.

The patient has come to see you on trust that you will guard their emotional and physical safety. This applies even if the patient's non-verbal communication is signalling a desire for greater intimacy. Sexual contact within a therapeutic relationship is unprofessional and potentially very harmful. It can be considered an abuse of trust and power, and you need to actively avoid placing yourself in such a situation.

Even allowing a new friendship to grow between yourself and the patient needs to be thought through very carefully, probably with the help of a supervisor. If a dual relationship is attempted the different boundaries between practitioner–patient and practitioner–friend will cause confusion. Some therapies have very strict codes of conduct around these issues; it would be better if they all had. The recommended time gap between knowing someone as a patient and forming a friendship or sexual relationship with them, is one year.

PROFESSIONAL BOUNDARIES

I remember going to a reflective practice conference in the 1990s and while talking to a doctor during the break time, I was startled to hear him say, 'We have practice meetings with the other consultants where we have a good laugh at what patients say about their illnesses.' Laughter is frequently used as a way of de-stressing for professionals who work regularly in traumatizing situations, such as fire-fighters, ambulance personnel or those who work in the emergency room. But to laugh at what the patient said is disrespectful and breaks the professional boundary. Paul E. McGhee (1996) has researched into the healing power of laughter and writes:

Laughing with [others] has a positive focus, characterized by support, caring, and empathy. Laughing at, on the other hand, generally communicates a sense of contempt and insensitivity, exclusion, one-upmanship, and even abuse. Laughing with focuses on the situation, while laughing at centres more around the person. (p.177)

Any notes, recordings or other information from a consultation should always be kept confidential and locked up between sessions. If you need to take a case to supervision, you should inform the patient and their name, address and any identifying details should be changed or simply omitted to maintain confidentiality. When you are with your supervisor or critical friend, remember to talk about all patients and other practitioners with respect. We can never really know the full story, but we can assume that everyone does the best they can within the circumstances.

Confidentiality extends to meeting your patient casually or accidentally outside of the clinic. You should never mention to any third party that your patient is on your books. It is up to the patient to reveal this or keep it private.

In the talking therapies such as homeopathy or counselling there should be no need for you to disclose your personal beliefs, issues or experiences to the patient. Physical therapies on the other hand, can proceed more smoothly if the practitioner chats lightly during the session about their garden, pet cat or the weather – unless the patient is clearly dozing or sleeping. Further disclosure would be unprofessional and you should not be talking about personal issues such as your hopes, needs or anxieties about your relationship, your children, your financial circumstances, or your career. This sort of disclosure shifts the relationship away from therapeutic towards friendship. It could even reverse the relationship so that the patient is forced into being the therapist listening to your problems.

TIME AND MONEY BOUNDARIES

In a short article written by my colleague, Caroline Schuck, and myself, we considered the boundaries of time and money as well as those of relationships. If the first consultation is much shorter than the advertised time, then the patient will feel they have been done a disservice. On the other hand, 'It may appear at first sight that giving the patient extra time for their money is a generosity' (Schuck and

Wood 2007). However, if the patient wasn't expecting more time, it can throw out the rest of their day, such as a mother needing to get to school on time to collect her children.

If you give or take extra time outside the working agreement, it can send mixed messages. It might lead the patient to think that other aspects of the working agreement do not need to be taken seriously or it might give the impression that you are always relaxed about time, and that it is okay for them to arrive late for appointments. Future appointments that are kept to time might feel too short for the patient.

Consider how you would feel if the patient decided to take more of your time than you had expected or intended, such as phoning you or texting you several times a day. Sooner or later you will become very irritated and uncaring. It is kinder to both you and your patient to set clear boundaries about how often they can contact you; and how often you will return their calls.

In the same way, undercharging or not charging for one aspect of the treatment gives mixed messages about the working agreement, and makes the patient feel awkward. Patients who are not charged can feel they are being put under an unfair obligation; or they feel embarrassed if their symptoms haven't got better; or guilty about trespassing on the practitioner's time. They might feel they have to return the favour by bringing flowers or baking a cake.

Students or beginner practitioners who give free appointments in order to get experience will not be taken seriously, unless they are working for a specific charity. Patients are more likely to arrive promptly for appointments that are booked in and will be charged for whether they arrive or not; they will have less commitment for an appointment that is not paid for.

How do you feel about receiving a tip or a thank-you bottle of wine? Accepting gifts from patients is permissible for some therapies, but transgresses boundaries in others. A patient who does favours for or gives presents to you might feel as if they are only saying thank you, but it can make subtle changes to your relationship with them. The patient may feel after giving you a gift that they have accrued extra credit with you. The gift might be unconsciously used as an insurance policy by the patient, giving them the unspoken rights to call upon you in any perceived emergency; rights which they wouldn't have had otherwise.

SETTING AND MAINTAINING BOUNDARIES

It is *always* the responsibility of the practitioner – not the patient – to set the practice boundaries. As practitioners, we can assume that the patient is adult, aware, intelligent and so on, but in terms of this relationship they have come for your help, expertise and professionalism because they are unwell. They are on your territory being treated by your therapy and it is your responsibility to make a working agreement that creates clear boundaries about relationships, professionalism, time and money.

The novice practitioner might ask: how do you hold to a boundary? The first step is to choose your boundaries by deciding exactly what you want in terms of practice hours, contact hours, fees, numbers and types of patient and so on. Decide these in detail, carefully thinking through issues like whether you want to be available at weekends, what are the different fee structures you might need, whether you want to treat children or whether you have accessibility for the disabled. You can include your proposed locum arrangements for when you are on holiday, and when you will or won't answer phone calls or texts. There are no right or wrong answers and you can choose exactly the practice you want.

Then you need to communicate all of these details to your patients. It might be easiest to put these on your website, but you might choose to hand them out as a fact-sheet or flyer to each patient. If you need to change them at any time, that's fine, just let your patients know.

To maintain your boundaries, try to be very clear about who you are when you are working. You are a qualified practitioner and you should be aiming to be a professional representative of your therapy. Take a few minutes to think about your journey to become a practitioner; the months or years of study, the hard-won skills, the enjoyment of working with people, the warmth you feel towards your patients and so on. Feel proud of your achievement, and give yourself respect.

Then consider professionalism across lawyers, accountants, bankers, teachers and so on. They all have clarity of purpose, integrity, dignity and self-respect, which is conveyed through their clothing, body language, facial expression, tone of voice and choice of words. You should feel like that.

Does that sound too difficult? Maybe your natural tendency is to be easy-going and have soft boundaries. Many practitioners have started out that way, and it feels wonderful to be generous towards your patients, but it doesn't pay off in the long run. Maybe your generosity is just another form of Rescuing the patient (see Chapter 3's section: 'The Drama Triangle'). Rescuing makes you feel good, but if it goes on for too long you will eventually become resentful and possibly blame the patient.

A newly registered practitioner asked for my help because she felt unable to build up her practice. She was meeting a lot of mothers in the playground after school and was using this as a way of talking about her therapy, hoping to get some new patients. Instead she found that she was giving away a lot of free advice, so much so that they did not need to come to see her professionally.

I explained to her that she would need much tighter boundaries to succeed, and if she wanted to give anything out in the playground, it should be business cards and flyers. The problem was that she wasn't used to having clear boundaries and it didn't come naturally to her. We decided that she would consciously invoke a separate persona to do this for her, as if she was acting a part or putting on her superwoman outfit. I suggested that she chose someone to copy, such as a schoolteacher or businesswoman. After several weeks of pretending to be more formal and boundaried than she would naturally be, she found that she had integrated boundaries into her thinking.

Setting the boundaries and creating a contracted relationship does not mean having rigid rules with no flexibility. Choosing the boundaries enables you to understand what suits you and your profession. It creates a framework which brings safety and security to both you and your patient. However within the chosen framework you can then renegotiate chosen aspects with an individual patient, making a temporary change of working agreement.

I asked a small group of experienced practitioners the following questions:

- Is your clinic room a neutral space, or does it reveal a lot about you?

- Do you give your patients time to express emotions if they need to?

- Do you keep to time when holding consultations/treatment sessions?

- Do you charge according to your advertised fees?

- Do you find yourself doing small favours for certain patients?

- Do you take dedicated time off for yourself?

In the discussion that arose from these questions, it was clear that the experienced practitioners were very confident about their boundaries although there was a big difference in where they set them. The more extrovert practitioners had wider boundaries, allowing the patients to have plenty of leeway – while the introverted practitioners had tighter, closer boundaries, allowing less flexibility. In answer to the first question, the extroverts allowed their personality to show through in the clinic room, while introverts preferred a more neutral space. All were very clear about what was permissible behaviour and all bent their own rules when they needed to.

COMPASSION WITHIN A FRAMEWORK

Santorelli (1999) asks us to remember our shared humanity within the practitioner–patient relationship. He does not suggest abandoning codes of conduct or medical ethics, but wants to introduce the time and space for compassion and connection. He writes:

> All too often the hard, impenetrable borders of this relationship are carved out of a process of identification that divides self and non-self into mutually exclusive entities. Unconsciously, this process winds up shaping the entire interaction. I am not suggesting that these roles are the same. They are not. But they are just that – roles. And behind these roles lies a much larger field, our shared humanness. This is all too easily and often forgotten. Yet it is the common ground of the entire relationship. (pp.61–62)

At first sight it might seem as if strong boundaries are at the polar opposite to compassion; but they are not. They clarify the ground rules allowing the practitioner to be honest about their needs. They create a framework in which the relationship can be genuine and the patient feels the freedom to fully express themselves. Once boundaries are in place you can consciously choose to deliberately bend or break them in certain circumstances.

◼ REFLECTIVE EXAMPLE

I graduated three years ago and I have concentrated on building up my practice through my website, my blog and generally networking. I have been quite casual about boundaries, because I had plenty of spare time. I've always told my patients to phone at any time if they had questions or concerns, and I got a lot of weekend calls. That didn't bother me. It felt good to have the interaction with the patients, I got updates on their health situations, and to be honest it made me feel busy. But now I'm finding it is too much. What should I do?

Brainstorm possible options

- Tell new patients they must only phone during weekdays up to 6.30pm, but allow old patients to continue phoning anytime. That would be favouring my old patients for their loyalty, but I don't really want any weekend calls.

- Tell all patients they must only phone during weekdays. That feels like nice firm boundaries, but what if they have a real emergency?

- Leave a message on my answerphone giving the number of someone they can phone at weekends. That should help them, but the other person might charge a lot.

- Tell all patients to phone during weekdays, and that they can phone me if it is an emergency over the weekend – but I will charge a lot. I'll charge double. I think if it is a real emergency, my patients will be grateful to speak to me rather than someone else and they won't mind paying double. If it's not an emergency they can wait until Monday.

Action plan

Do a mail out this week explaining my decision to charge double. Ask my friend to check the wording if necessary. Review results in three weeks.

Three weeks later

Surprisingly I got a lot of positive feedback about my decision to charge double for weekend emergency calls. I was half expecting to lose some patients as it is a big price rise. To my surprise, a couple of them said they had wondered when I was going to put my prices up, and they still felt it was an excellent service. Wow! I hadn't expected that. Patient X e-mailed me to say she felt a lot better now that I had clarified my fees and hours. She said that she had phoned me several times at weekends, but it felt uncomfortable and she felt guilty doing it.

Nobody has had an emergency so far; and it feels blissful to have my weekends back to myself again!

EXERCISE: OTHER PEOPLE'S BOUNDARIES

Think back to a situation where you were the patient and you went to see a doctor, a therapist, a dentist or any other practitioner.

Were the boundaries clear? Did you feel safe with this practitioner?

If the boundaries were very clear with this practitioner, spend some time identifying what they did to make it clear to you, and how this felt.

If the boundaries were not clear, write about what happened within your relationship with the practitioner. In particular, focus on your feelings.

EXERCISE: REVIEW YOUR BOUNDARIES

Take the time to review your boundaries. Do they really suit you? Have they been explained to your patients, where appropriate? Are they effective?

You could do this as a drawing or painting allowing yourself complete freedom of expression. Take a few minutes before you start to sit quietly, relax your body and just listen to your breathing. You don't need to change your breathing, just be aware of how you are breathing, and allow all other thoughts to fade into the background. When you have quietened your mind somewhat, collect up your paints, pens and paper. Represent yourself as a figure, a shape or just a colour and choose very carefully where on the page you place yourself. Add your patients as a group or as individuals, your professional association, your clinic space and your family, friends and colleagues – or any combination of these. Finally put in the boundary lines, choosing carefully what sort of line it would be: thick, thin, broken, open, incomplete, intact? And what colour it would be: black as a legal document, red as a warning sign, turquoise as a protection, pink as undecided?

Leave your drawing or painting for a few hours or a day and then come back to it and analyse what you see, or take it into supervision. Your supervisor, peers or critical friend don't need to analyse it. They can just give you feedback on what they observe and gently question you about it. Usually with this sort of reflection, some of your unconscious thoughts and feelings become represented in the picture. On one level there is what you thought you were representing, but you may well find some new connections on carefully observing your picture for a second time.

EXERCISE: MINDFUL BOUNDARIES

Sit somewhere where you can be comfortable and quiet, either cross-legged on the floor or in a chair with your feet on the floor. Take some time being aware of your body, and how it is being supported by the chair or the floor. Notice your breathing, and without judging or trying to change it, simply hold your attention on the air going in and out of your nostrils and down into your lungs. Stay with it for a few minutes.

Then visualize that you are in a large green space that is enclosed, such as a big garden with an old wooden fence and a gate, or a field with an ancient hedge and a large five-bar gate, or a wide park with painted railings and a tall gate. In your imagination, quietly walk around the perimeter of the green space until you come to the gate. It is your green space and you can open the gate easily. Without thinking too much, allow your mind to quietly dwell on what it feels like to have a green space with an enclosing barrier. Stay with the feeling, breathing the fresh air and quietly, slowly looking around. When you are ready, come back to the present. Make a few notes in your journal.

Chapter 10

SOLVING ETHICAL DILEMMAS

Ethics are a way of defining standards for moral conduct. They identify what is acceptable or unacceptable behaviour within the community. Moral values take us beyond the need for instant gratification, such as that felt by the newborn baby who is hungry. They remind us to stop and consider the impact our behaviour will have on our future selves or on other people.

A code of ethics is a set of principles that guide the moral conduct of a specific community, establishing common standards and expectations. They are created and defined by the organizations or associations that represent each profession and every practitioner within the organization agrees to abide by them. Codes of ethics confirm the boundary between acceptable and unacceptable behaviour for the benefit of the patient, the practitioner and the therapy itself. They help us do the right thing even if no one is looking.

WHY DO WE NEED CODES OF ETHICS?

A code of ethics both defines and sets the standards for a profession. It clarifies boundaries, expectations and moral values. This is especially important within healthcare where one person is not-well and the other person is well. (The practitioner assumes the status of wellness during the consultation, whatever their personal health at other times.)

A typical code of ethics begins with definitions to clarify the aims of the therapy and its philosophy or underlying principles. It highlights the values of the profession, such as acting independently, legally, safely, respectfully, with accountability and integrity. It reminds practitioners about legal considerations and it provides a document that patients or the general public can refer to.

BOX 10.1 CODES OF ETHICS MIGHT INCLUDE...

- the aims of the therapy
- the philosophy or underlying principles of the therapy
- the values that promote a good working relationship
- accountability to the profession and to the public
- integrity of the practitioner and the profession
- legal considerations.

Some of the more common values that are seen in different codes of ethics are setting up a working agreement, creating clear boundaries and respecting the patient's need for safety, confidentiality, dignity and autonomy. The first two of these I have discussed at length already (Chapters 4 and 9) but the others are worth briefly revisiting.

SAFETY

Safety has been discussed in terms of the working agreement (see Chapter 4) and boundaries (see Chapter 9). The patient also needs to be physically safe according to the law, so the consulting room needs safe access, safe equipment and even safe toys for the children. It is up to you to decide how to interpret this. Alternative remedies that are prescribed should not conflict with medical prescriptions and the patient should consult with their doctor before making any changes to their medicine or dosage.

Emotionally, they need the safety of confidentiality, and compassion. If they become emotional during the session, you need to give them enough time to calm down before going home. There are several ways of doing this. If you are a body-worker you could choose a soothing, comforting touch for the last five minutes. If it has been a long talking session, such as the homeopathic consultation, you can ask a few very basic, easy-to-answer questions towards the end of the session. You can offer them the bathroom before they leave. If the patient is very emotional and beyond any of these strategies, you might inquire whether there is anyone who can assist them on the journey home, or who will be at home to support them.

Another aspect of ethical safety is that you should be competent in your therapy, having received appropriate training in theory and adequate experience in practice; and you need to have a commitment to CPD (Continuing Professional Development).

CONFIDENTIALITY

Confidentiality for the patient means both during the consultation and afterwards. Your patient ought to be able to talk freely without being overheard or overlooked. After the consultation, you should put the case notes in a safe place where they will not be seen by anyone. If the case needs to be shown to your supervisor, or details sent to their GP, you should explain this to the patient. Even then, the personal details should not be revealed to the supervisor (the name, address, phone numbers or profession). If you want to use your patient's case notes for teaching, advertising or publishing, you need to get their consent in writing and reassure them that personal details will not be revealed.

Having said this, confidentiality can never be absolute, because at times it conflicts with safety, such as when the patient is suicidal, plans harm to others, or who is a child that is being abused. In these sorts of circumstances you might be neglecting your duty of care if you placed the need for confidentiality above that of safety. The law of the land has to always be considered above any individual code of ethics.

DIGNITY

The patient should be allowed to retain their dignity throughout the consultation and treatment. The consultation part of the session should be done with both practitioner and patient sitting where they can see each other and have eye contact on a similar level. A patient lying on a treatment couch, puts themselves in the practitioner's hands to have a treatment like a massage or acupuncture session. But if they are being questioned, they are at a disadvantage if they are lying on the couch. To talk about themselves they need more equality of body language, such as both people sitting in chairs of equal height with eye contact. If the patient has to get undressed for the treatment, they should be able to do this in privacy, either behind a screen or left alone in the consulting room for a few minutes.

Physically, certain areas of the body are private and should be respected as such. Mentally and emotionally, most people keep some information private, to be revealed only in times of complete trust. A consultation is not an interrogation, and even if the practitioner suspects there is more to the story than the patient is ready to reveal, their only choice is to wait.

AUTONOMY

Where possible, you should respect the patient's autonomy. This means they should have the right to make their own decisions and act on them independently – providing they don't impinge on other people's autonomy or safety. However to do this they need to be mature enough to make informed choices, and parents or carers may have to make decisions for children, the elderly, the sick or the disabled. You should give patients enough information so that they can make an informed choice about their side of the treatment agreement. For example, they can choose the time and regularity of the appointments, within the practitioner's own boundary of working certain hours. Respecting the patient's autonomy means having a clear contract or working agreement (see Chapter 4).

ETHICAL CONFLICTS

Most codes of ethics have a strong common sense aspect, although maybe some go into too much detail. They are there to protect you as well as the patient and the profession as a whole. Most of them are easy to comply with as you just need to set up a protocol in your working practice and follow it. However, every so often an issue arises that causes a moral dilemma and the code of ethics has to be examined in more detail. Weighing up the ethics can help you navigate the grey area between right and wrong.

Ethical conflicts arise all the time in the form of philosophical questions that cannot be answered easily. Should you as a practitioner help everyone who comes to your clinic, equally? Presumably they are paying the same fee, unless they are a child, and they deserve an equal opportunity for healing. If one patient can be healed easily, but another needs three times as much time and effort on behalf of the practitioner, where is the equality? The time-consuming patient deserves healing as much as the other one, but if working to achieve this has a knock-on effect of exhausting the practitioner, then other patients will suffer (see Figure 10.1).

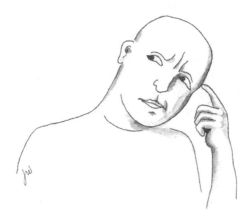

FIGURE 10.1: WEIGH UP EACH ETHICAL DILEMMA

In practice there are regular ethical conflicts but most of these are small enough that the practitioner can quickly resolve them without help. This could be the child who arrives hungry and irritable after school; food and drink are not allowed in the clinic, but you know the child will not cooperate without a snack. You might resolve this by directing the mother to somewhere where the child can eat the snack and return within ten minutes. Or you might spread out newspaper to protect the new carpet while the child eats in the clinic room.

One way that ethical conflicts can arise is when the patient cannot communicate easily for themselves, such as the elderly, the disabled, babies or young children. Carers or relatives will have to be present in the consultation which can compromise confidentiality and autonomy.

A young mother came to see me, because she wanted me to use remedies to dry up her milk so that she could stop breastfeeding. Her mother-in-law had come to stay, and told her that she was continuing breastfeeding for too long and that she should stop. I asked her about her views on breastfeeding, and she said that she had enjoyed it and the baby had put on weight. However, she felt convinced by her mother-in-law's arguments. I suggested a breastfeeding counsellor, but she refused. I told her that I would study the case and send my prescription to her later that day. My ethical dilemma was over who should benefit from this prescription. If my remedy stopped the milk, then the mother-in-law would benefit, and if it enabled the milk to continue, the baby would benefit. What would suit the young mother who was after all, my patient? She wanted both a happy mother-in-law and a happy baby. How did I feel about suppressing a natural and healthy process?

What would you have done with this ethical conflict? There is no easy answer. Whatever you decide in these sorts of cases, it is a good policy to keep notes on the advice you gave to the patient as well as the treatment you chose for them. In the above case, I noted that I asked her about her own views about breastfeeding and I recommended she visit a breastfeeding counsellor.

Ethical conflicts can arise because your own personal, social or religious values don't blend comfortably with your professional code of ethics. A student came to see me because she felt she couldn't recover from a broken relationship. After a long and tearful session, she revealed that the relationship had been with her college tutor, and I suddenly realized that I knew who she was talking about. Working in the same college, I knew that having a relationship with a student was against the tutor's and my code of ethics. Should I break my patient's confidence by exposing her lover? Probably not. Should I persuade her to expose him? Again, probably not, because it would open up all of her wounds again. But if I don't do anything about it, I'm left with the uncomfortable knowledge that a fellow tutor got away with something unethical – and for all I knew he might do it again.

Conflict can arise if you're trying to practise within two codes of ethics. One of my colleagues was working in a voluntary capacity to help rehabilitate drug users. The patients were only allowed onto the program if they had given up using drugs. A young woman came for several sessions and was becoming a lot more positive and healthy. One day she arrived at a consultation, clearly under the influence of drugs. The practitioner knew that he should report this, but if he did, the young woman would be thrown off the program and would probably not return. Reporting the young woman would mean breaking confidentiality – which was against the practitioner's professional code of conduct but a regular part of the code belonging to the rehabilitation centre. He wanted to negotiate with the young woman to stop the drugs immediately so that she could stay on the program, but that could risk his integrity as a volunteer, and possibly the integrity of the program itself.

We can look at this case through the values considered previously: those of a working agreement with clear boundaries and respect for the patient's safety, confidentiality, dignity and autonomy.

- A working agreement with clear boundaries was in place: the program clearly states that no one on drugs should enter the program. Both practitioner and patient understood this.

- Autonomy: the young woman has made her own decision to go back to drugs. The practitioner wants her to immediately stop so she can stay on the program.

- Safety: the patient's decision conflicts with her safety and her health; if the practitioner decides to go on helping her, he has the patient's safety in mind.

- Confidentiality: following the program's code of ethics, the practitioner should break confidentiality and report the young woman. If the practitioner followed his own code of ethics, he would keep confidentiality and negotiate with the woman to stop the drugs and return to the program.

- Dignity: if the young woman returns to the program, she gains some self-respect.

PRINCIPLES FROM MORAL PHILOSOPHY

Tim Bond (1993), writing in *Standards and Ethics for Counselling in Action* looked at four principles of moral philosophy in terms of building a code of ethics (p.33). These have wonderful sounding names that roll off the tongue. *Beneficence* means a commitment to benefit the client and its opposite, *non-malificence* means to consciously avoid harming the client. *Justice* means having a fair distribution of services within the society, and *autonomy* means self-government (see Box 10.2). However, Bond (1993) reminds us, 'These principles do not always work in harmony' (p.34).

Returning to the case of the young woman on the drug program, we could argue either way for beneficence and non-malificence. How could we say what will achieve the greatest good in this case? Is it better for the practitioner to rescue her, or is it better for her to learn the hard way and take responsibility? Which will cause the least harm? To throw the woman off the program, or risk having the practitioner removed from the program?

BOX 10.2 PRINCIPLES FROM MORAL PHILOSOPHY

- Beneficence: what will achieve the greatest good?
- Non-malificence: what will cause the least harm?
- Justice: what will be fairest?
- Respect for autonomy: what is the individual's choice?
- These apply to you as well.

It is interesting to look at justice. Fairness towards the young woman suggests that the practitioner should give her a chance to rehabilitate, while fairness towards the others on the program demands that all similar cases get the same treatment. But if the drug program condoned one slip-up for everyone, are they then colluding with drug addiction? Allowing the young woman to stay on the program even though she has taken drugs recently is unfair to the program itself because both practitioner and patient are cheating the system (albeit for a good cause).

Then consider autonomy, which applies to everyone in the case. This allows both practitioner and the young woman to make their own decisions. In terms of the Drama Triangle, the practitioner wants to Rescue the woman who appears to be in Victim mode, helplessly travelling towards a life of crime, prostitution and drugs.

In this case you might feel that the pendulum is swinging towards negotiating with this young woman to give her a last chance, although there are still several arguments against it. This may be as good as it gets. Working with the aid of moral values or Bond's principles from moral philosophy (or both) will certainly help you clarify your thinking, even if some areas aren't working in harmony with the rest.

Another way of looking at ethics is to ask yourself these three questions:

- Would your course of action be recommended by others or would you recommend it? (Universality)

- Would you tell other practitioners, or publish your course of action? (Publicity)

- Would you do the same for others in the same situation or for a famous or influential client? (Justice)

Looking at the case above, it's easy to see that if the woman gets a second chance, it is not something you would want to recommend for all of the people at the program, and you would probably not publish your course of action. You would not recommend it to others and others would not recommend it to you. This time the pendulum has swung away from trying to help the young woman.

ETHICS ARE EASY, ETHICAL CONFLICTS ARE COMPLEX

Working with ethics is relatively easy, when there is just one code of ethics and you're simply asking a question, 'Is this ethical?' You can be in the place of the unprejudiced observer, adult or leveller and when you check the code of ethics you will get a simple answer yes or no. Working with ethical conflict on the other hand means that the answers will not be clear, and it will be more difficult to be unprejudiced; your own preferences, instinct and intuition start to play a part. All you can do is weigh up as many different factors as you can and make an informed choice.

REFLECTIVE EXAMPLE

A man of 70 came to see me today because his consultant was seriously concerned about the onset of gangrene in his feet. He was advised that he had to stop smoking immediately or he might end up losing his legs. He decided he would prefer to continue smoking, a lifelong habit that he couldn't do without, and he wanted me to see what I could do about the gangrene. I tried my best to listen to him respectfully, but all the while I was conscious of my own sense of shock that he could not give up smoking even at the risk of losing his legs. I listened carefully to his story and I asked questions to understand him better. I told him that I would prefer to make a prescription to boost his health generally this week and if he would book an appointment for the following week, I would prescribe more specifically for the gangrene. This was a reasonable treatment plan, but I chose it mainly because it bought me time to think carefully about the ethics of this situation. However, it didn't give him much room for negotiation.

Respect for individual *autonomy* means accepting the patient's choice. This man's choice is that he should continue smoking at the risk of losing his legs. Maybe he just can't face considering what it would be like to lose his legs, whereas he's got a very clear idea of what it would be like to lose his cigarettes. He said that he didn't think he would live much longer anyway and he might as well enjoy his life. He was definitely committed to his decision not to give up cigarettes. Maybe he thought the consultant's view was just an idle threat. Providing he is not being delusional and has good mental health, I should accept his choice and try to help him.

Beneficence means a commitment to benefiting the client or patient. What will be in the patient's best interest? What would increase their health? As far as I can see all research suggests that smoking does not increase health and most often decreases health. If he could come to me regularly over the course of a month, I might be able to help with the gangrene (there is no saying for sure). But increased health of his feet would encourage him to continue smoking – which will not benefit him in the long term.

Non-malificence means avoiding harm to the client or patient. If I was able to help him with the gangrene it might only be temporary relief before getting worse again. Enabling him to continue smoking is colluding with his view that cigarettes can do little harm. I think that following this path would be harmful to the patient.

Justice should include the whole community. If I cured his other health problems, which would enable him to continue smoking, does that mean I'm condoning smoking? Would I encourage younger members of his family to take up smoking; or would I happily treat someone else so that they could continue smoking? My answer is most certainly not. This feels like an abuse of my skills and knowledge.

Justice could also include the necessity for transparency with the patient, which is something that I didn't do so well. I did not want to threaten the patient the same way that the consultant had done, in the manner of, 'If you don't stop smoking I can't help you.' I negotiated that I would treat him constitutionally this week and specifically next week, and this was professional in itself, but includes an element of collusion if I'm prepared to work specifically on the gangrene.

Finally I can apply these to me, because I also deserve autonomy, beneficence, non-malificence and justice. It was good that I respected the patient's choice, but that doesn't mean I should be the practitioner who condones his smoking. I could have simply told him that I was unable to prescribe for him on an ethical basis. To make it easier for him, I could have told him I was prejudiced against smoking and would end up giving him a lecture the same as his consultant had done. That is treating him as an Adult, but warning him that one of my options is to act out the Critical Parent.

EXERCISE: ETHICAL PROBLEM-SOLVING

Using your reflective journal, write a brief written description of your ethical dilemma in order to clarify the main points. Decide whether it is the patient's dilemma, or your own. Then do some research into any guidelines that you can access, such as your professional code of ethics, and any laws that are applicable, such as health and safety, child protection or data protection. Now you are in a position to brainstorm all possible courses of action.

EXERCISE: EVALUATING AFTER YOUR DECISION

Think back to when you had an ethical dilemma, and evaluate the outcome. What can you learn from it? Is it something that you can look back on and feel that you took a good decision in the circumstances? (I suggest you will complicate things if you use the words 'right decision' about an ethical dilemma.)

Would your course of action be recommended by others or would you recommend it? (Universality)

Would you tell other practitioners, or publish your course of action? (Publicity)

Would you do the same for others in the same situation or for a famous or influential client? (Justice)

If you find that you have come to a different conclusion in looking at your ethical dilemma through these three questions, compared to your decision in the past, then don't be hard on yourself. Ethical dilemmas can be very tough and working through any sort of question-and-answer format takes time. Accept that you have learned from the experience, you did the best you could at the time and maybe you'll do it differently next time.

EXERCISE: HOW DO YOU FEEL ABOUT YOUR CODE OF ETHICS?

Does your therapy have a code of ethics? Have you read it recently? Do you feel that it fairly represents your therapy and the values that are important to you?

Make some notes in your journal about how you perceive your code of ethics. If you don't like them, how would you change them?

Chapter 11

FINISHING THE SESSION AND CLOSURE

Closure is a psychological term used when someone gains a resolution to a significant event or a relationship – and they feel satisfied with that conclusion. Sometimes this is a matter of finding some missing information when the issue was previously confused. Closure can also mean ending or finishing, such as at the end of each session with the patient or at the end of a series of sessions.

FINISHING A SESSION

The process of negotiation and planning for the future (see Chapter 8) frequently becomes interwoven with closure. They have been written as separate stages for the sake of clarification and mindfulness.

For the patient, the finishing process allows them a little breathing space between the intensity of the consultation or treatment and the journey home. This acts in the same way as the introduction, which was a breathing space between the arrival and the consultation. It gives the patient the opportunity of closing down any emotional and intellectual barriers that were opened up during the consultation (see Box 11.1).

The patient has probably lost sense of time while they were having a session with you, so it is helpful if you can warn them, 'We are coming towards the end of the session' or 'We have five minutes left.' In the remaining time, you can ask them if there is anything else they wanted to say and whether they have any questions. You might want to give them the opportunity to phone you when they get home if they think of anything else, but in most cases this would be opening up your boundaries, which is not recommended.

If a patient has had an emotional session they need to have the opportunity to calm down and return to normal before they leave.

Sometimes you can leave some innocent questions such as date of birth and address to the end of the consultation. These will act as calming questions. In other cases you might need to ask the patient if they want to sit quietly for a few minutes, or use the bathroom, or have a glass of water. Occasionally after a healing session or after a guided meditation, the patient is left feeling spacey, distant or dazed. The quickest way to get them to come back into their bodies is to offer something to eat or drink. A glass of water will do.

BOX 11.1 FINISHING THE SESSION

- Warn the patient that you're nearly at the end of the session.
- Help calm an emotional or upset patient.
- Offer a dazed or sleepy patient a glass of water.
- Ask them if there's anything more they want to say.
- Ask them if they have any questions.
- Thank the patient for being cooperative.
- Confirm the treatment plan.
- Book in the next appointment and take the fees.
- See the patient to the door.

From the patient's point of view, they have spent some or all of the time with you trying to explain themselves. This is a difficult task when talking to a comparative stranger and they may be left with a sense that they haven't described themselves well enough. You might have experienced this yourself. Think back to a session you had with a doctor, dentist or alternative practitioner. Choose a session where a lot of information was passed to and from the practitioner. What were your feelings on walking away from the session? Did you feel some frustration that you had not been able to explain yourself well enough? Did you have the thoughts, 'Oh, I wish I had said this or that'?

Not everyone talks easily about themselves, but you can be sure that the larger proportion of your patients have tried hard to cooperate, whether successfully or otherwise. After all, they are paying for your treatment and want to benefit from it. I suggest they deserve praise and thanks for telling their story and sharing the responsibility for healing. Some patients might have the delusion that they made a fool of themselves in crying or talking too much. They need your reassurance that showing emotion is perfectly acceptable and that it is a frequent reaction to the treatment or (depending on the therapy) that it will confirm the treatment plan. Your job at the moment is to help the patient feel comfortable with what has happened during the session, and prepare them to face the outside world again (see Figure 11.1).

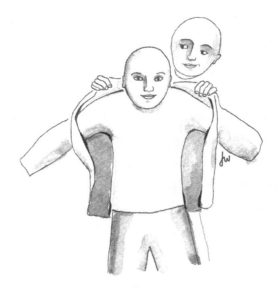

FIGURE 11.1: HELP THE PATIENT PREPARE FOR THE OUTSIDE WORLD

The final part of finishing a session is the administration. If the practitioner is self-employed they may have to change roles at this point and become their own practice manager. For some practitioners this is surprisingly difficult, coming straight after a session with the patient where they were using either touch or words to become close and familiar. It is as if they are trying to jump from the role of gentle healer into the role of hard-headed accountant or worse still, bailiff. The gap between these roles feels too great, making the practitioner awkward or clumsy when it comes to administration. For others, there is less of a gap between the roles. In the session they are the self-employed practitioner and afterwards they are the administrator.

If you find you have a problem with doing administration and don't have a receptionist to take over, I suggest that you consciously change roles by using a simple ritual that could be done in front of the patient. Rituals can be made out of moving into another room, washing your hands, stripping the paper off the couch, closing your books, putting all the notes back into the folder or simply picking up your diary to book the next appointment. Do this simple task holding the awareness that in this moment, now, you have no role, you are simply being. Do the task mindfully and when it is complete, assume the other role. A one-minute ritual like this also indicates non-verbally to the patient that the session has ended.

Administration includes taking the fees and booking the next appointment. It might also include a confirmation of the treatment plan, although this might have been done earlier, depending upon your therapy. Before the patient leaves, have a quick check to see if they have forgotten anything.

HOLIDAY COVER

All practitioners need time away from work, the same as everyone else. It is an important part of their self-care. However patients do not choose when they get ill, so you need to make arrangements for them while you are away. If you take a regular block of time out, such as a month every August or the two weeks that your children are on holiday every Christmas, then this could be written into your terms and conditions, either given out as a flyer or on your website. Whenever you take time off, you should put brief messages on phone and e-mail, saying when you'll be back and who patients can contact in the meantime.

As a homeopath, I always asked a colleague to locum for me while I was away, but most of the time the patients just needed reassurance and the locum did not need to prescribe anything. Sometimes they would send the patient to their local doctor. If they did have to make a homeopathic prescription, the patient would pay them directly. On the other hand, my acupuncturist would go to China for a month every summer, and she arranged for her locum to use her clinic and have access to the patient's notes (with their consent), so they could have regular treatments.

A patient who tries to contact their practitioner but gets no reply from their messages left on phone or e-mail will start to get irritable if they imagine the practitioner has no sense of responsibility; or anxious if they imagine the practitioner is unwell. When they find out later that they have just been on holiday there might be a sense of betrayal and abandonment.

The bottom line is that it doesn't matter how you choose to arrange your holidays, but it is professional to let your patients know how long you will be away for, when you'll be back and what you suggest they do in the meantime if they have a problem. This can all be on your e-mail and voicemail out-of-office notifications.

If you are unwell, you need to make a decision about whether to cancel your appointments for that day or for that week, or whether you can carry on as usual. It is your duty of care to inform the patient of any cancellations as far in advance as possible, and to arrange for new appointments. For many alternative practices, sending the patient to another practitioner to cover a missed appointment is not feasible. Timing and location might not match up easily and the urgent transfer of patient notes could be very difficult.

PATIENTS WHO DO NOT RETURN

Closure means being at peace with the patient's decision to leave. With some patients, leaving is clearly the right decision as they were not comfortable with your therapy or they were not making any progress. With other patients there is a sort of open diary agreement. They are not coming for appointments at the moment, but you have arranged that they will return when they need to, perhaps in six months' time. Some patients return once a year for a check up (like a regular service on your car). With these patients you do not need closure.

A final session with a patient who has indicated they are leaving would be the ideal, because you can do a review of your work together. This only takes five or ten minutes and allows both of you to say what you have gained from the consultations and the treatments. It is a good idea to return to your first set of notes from the first consultation, and remind the patient of the symptoms they had when they first arrived. This really clarifies for the patient what has been improved or cured as well as which symptoms are still outstanding.

However, when patients leave abruptly even though you felt they were making good progress, it can be very confusing. Maybe they didn't perceive the improvement that you saw, maybe they were impatient for a faster rate of cure, maybe they found someone else who was cheaper or closer to home or maybe they have returned to orthodox medicine. It can be difficult to sit with not knowing why your patient left, and sometimes it creates feelings of disappointment, abandonment, guilt or frustration. You might feel that you could have helped this patient given a bit more time or you might feel guilty that you did not get them better. It might hurt your professional pride, or might make a dent in your income. You might find you are asking yourself questions such as 'What did I do wrong?' Without closure with the patient, these questions could be left hanging and potentially could eat into your self-confidence if you answer them in the negative.

The aim of closure in this context is for you to feel comfortable about the patient leaving, without judging them or yourself. It would be a courtesy from them to let you know they are leaving, but they don't have to give their reasons. It is the perfect place for you to practise compassion towards them and to yourself. I suggest that you either reflect in your journal, or you reflect with a critical friend or supervisor. You could begin with writing two lists, *What I did well* and *What I didn't do so well*, in order to get a balanced view of all your work with this patient. Maybe you did make some mistakes and it is time to acknowledge them, but it is also time to praise yourself for what you did well. You might want to analyse your relationship with this patient. Does it fit into any of the relationship patterns written about in Chapter 3? Do you see a Drama Triangle going on or any of the three ego states coming into play?

You can write an unsent letter in your journal to the patient. Write directly to the patient, telling them your views. You can reveal all your emotions because this letter is in your journal and will not actually be sent. Finish your letter with a list of at least six things that you appreciated about this patient and wish them good health for the future.

I did this exercise with a practitioner who was very fed up with a patient leaving her. This patient had always pushed the boundaries and demanded extra attention, so in some ways it was a relief when she moved on to another practitioner. But she left owing money and the manner of her leaving was abrupt and unpleasant. The practitioner started off the unsent letter with her irritation and anger, and then I asked her to feel a little compassion and write about what was appealing in that patient. She wrote about the patient's courage in the face of difficult decisions – and then began to wonder if the patient had found the process of leaving her difficult, and whether she had simply been clumsy in her farewells out of embarrassment. The practitioner decided to write a brief and compassionate goodbye letter that she would send, enclosing an invoice for the money outstanding.

Another way of reviewing what happened with a patient is to try to understand them from the inside, by miming them or talking like them. While you are in role get your critical friend (or your journal) to ask you why you stopped coming to clinics. You might find that you do know the answer unconsciously, and when you role-play the patient it is revealed.

If the patient has died, you might want to do a small ritual, such as lighting a candle or writing a card (sent or unsent) to say goodbye. Write in your journal a list of what you appreciated about them, and what you will miss now they have gone. Send them your blessings. You may or may not feel it is appropriate to attend the funeral of a patient. If you have treated someone for a long time you will have come to know them very well and going to the funeral will help your grieving process, providing it does not add to the grief of the family. Maybe they did not know the deceased was coming to see you.

Finish your journal entry with some self-compassion, either spoken or written. This is a process of comforting yourself like a mother comforts her baby. Stroke your skin or hold your hand above your heart area, and tell yourself gentle, soothing words like, 'All practitioners lose patients sometimes, it's not just me, it is part of being a practitioner, I don't need to take it personally, I do very well with most of my patients, other practitioners have difficult cases and this was one of mine. I felt privileged to be working with this patient, and I felt I was providing some relief. I learned a lot and I'm deeply sorry that they have passed away. Sadly, it is one of the drawbacks of working with the elderly.'

As the last step of closure with a patient who is leaving your practice, I recommend writing a short letter or e-mail to the patient which you *will* send to them. Keep it very brief, along the lines of, 'Thank you and best wishes.' For example, 'Thank you for telling me you are leaving and I am sorry that I could not do more for you. My very best wishes for your future health.' Do not include any specific explanations or apologies and do not ask them why they are leaving. Keep it very general and re-read your letter several times to make sure no bitterness has entered into it. Write from the role of Adult and remember that the leaving patient needs compassion as well. There is an added advantage that if you are sweet natured when they leave, they might come back to you in the future, or they might send one of their friends to come to you. Keep a copy of this letter in their file.

There are some occasions where it is necessary to make a termination agreement with the patient. This might happen if the patient is mentally ill, when it is practical to clarify when treatment comes to a stop. It also might happen if you, yourself, are ill. You don't need to explain yourself or give reasons for finishing treatment. You can simply say, 'I'm no longer in a position to help you.' You can write this in a letter to them, and keep a copy in your file, or you can make a written agreement that they have to sign, saying that the therapeutic relationship has come to an end.

IN CONCLUSION

If a patient only comes for one treatment and then disappears, it can be frustrating for the practitioner. There is a delicate balance whether you contact them to find out what happened, or whether you respect their silence and wait and see. If the patient has been with you for some time and is now leaving you because they feel so much better, you might feel a small sadness at their loss coupled with a thrill of satisfaction at their improvement. If the patient leaves because they no longer want to work with you, it can give you a sense of disappointment, frustration or failure. It is the same when a patient dies. In these cases, you need to do some self-reflection of your work with them, praising yourself for what you did well, understanding what you could have done better and comforting yourself for not being perfect.

▐ REFLECTIVE EXAMPLE

Patient X phoned up today completely out of the blue, and said, 'I have decided to move on.' I had no idea what she was talking about, and said something neutral in order to encourage her to say more. She said, 'I thought it was about time to find someone with a fresh approach, who would see everything through new eyes.' I still didn't get it, and mumbled, 'I'm not sure...' Finally she said something about her new practitioner, and with a shock I realized that this was a courtesy call to say she was leaving me as a practitioner. I thanked her and said something about it being okay if the new practitioner wanted to contact me about the notes.

What were my feelings?

When I put the phone down, I was feeling shocked and numb. Then I felt really upset. She had been coming to see me for a couple of years and the decision to leave was completely unexpected. Even when she was telling me she was leaving I didn't understand it. She's not from the UK, and I think that sometimes she translates phrases literally from her own language which makes strange idioms in English.

Evaluation: what was good about treating her?

She was lively and vivacious and had a good sense of humour, and I enjoyed her appointments. She was my 'kudos patient' who boosted my self-confidence. She was loyal to me over two years and always paid on time.

Evaluation: what was not so good about treating her?

She talked too much and frequently overstayed her appointment. I think I was a little bit in awe of her and didn't always keep to my boundaries. She didn't always follow my instructions because she was so busy. Sometimes it was very difficult to make a good prescription for her and although I helped her quite a lot, I never completely cured her.

Analysis

My colleague describes this as the 'Dear John' moment; the letter that John gets from his girlfriend to say that she doesn't want to see him any more. It's the shock of rejection when you don't see it coming.

Another cause of my shock was because I was proud of this patient. She is a big name, she is famous. I kept total confidentiality and didn't even tell my supervisor, but it gave me a nice warm feeling inside that she should come to visit me as a practitioner.

Conclusion

I think the main problem was that my pride was hurt. I called her my 'kudos patient'.

What should I do now?

I will write her a little note to say all the best for the future and let me know if there is anything I can help with. I can say that I enjoyed working with her. I can let go with love. I will spend some time tomorrow appreciating all my other patients. I was beginning to feel that patient X was special and more interesting than the other patients, and that was my mistake. All of my patients are interesting and lovely people, they've all got stories to tell, they are all special.

EXERCISE: WRITING YOUR GOODBYE LETTER

Practise writing a letter or e-mail that you will be able to use if any patient decides to leave you. Make it a short letter and include best wishes for the future, and thank them for coming to see you. Consider what else you might want to say, such as offering help to the new practitioner, or suggesting to the patient that you are available if they want to come back in the future. This is not an easy letter to write, which is why you are practising it now. If you start off with creating a standard farewell letter, you can personalize it as you need to when it comes to a real case.

EXERCISE: LEAVING A PRACTITIONER

Think of any times that you have left a practitioner, whether it is the doctor, dentist, alternative practitioner or even your hairdresser. How often have you phoned, e-mailed or written to tell the practitioner that you were leaving? How often have you told yourself that you ought to tell them but never quite got round to it? Reflect on this. Was it simply your bad manners that prevented you from letting them know or were there other reasons?

How would you have felt if after three or six months your practitioner wrote to you to ask how you're getting on, or sent you a questionnaire on patient satisfaction levels after treatment? Under what conditions would you be happy to give feedback to the practitioner that you left?

Write some notes in your self-reflective journal, and consider if any of the answers apply to you in your role of practitioner.

EXERCISE: APPRECIATING YOUR PATIENT

Your first reaction after a patient passes away or leaves you abruptly for any other reason, might be irritation, frustration, anxiety, guilt, or abandonment. You might want to blame yourself for being an ineffective practitioner, or blame the patient for being unreliable. After this initial reaction, take some time to appreciate this patient, working with your reflective journal.

Make a list of what you appreciated about the patient. They can be very small things, such as the patient always arrived on time, they made a referral to you, they had a pleasant sounding voice or a beautiful smile, they were interesting to talk to or they were very receptive of your treatments. Then make a second list of all the things you have learned from treating this patient, like you had to do extra research into their case or they presented new challenges that you hadn't come across before. Add as much as you can to both lists and fully appreciate the patient for what they were and what they contributed to your life. Do not write down any of the exasperations or failures that they contributed to, just appreciate.

Chapter 12

SELF-CARE FOR THE PRACTITIONER

Working in a caring profession, listening to other people's stories of trauma, illness, disease, fear or unhappiness, can make the practitioner susceptible to compassion fatigue, vicarious trauma and burnout. This means that practitioners have a responsibility for their own self-care, because they cannot care for others if they are run down or burnt out. It might be that some practitioners neglect this responsibility out of egotism or naivety. Maybe a lifetime's habit of caring for others makes it seem selfish to take time off; or maybe they need a full appointments diary for the income. Perhaps they are simply hard task masters for themselves. Practitioners can be good at recommending their patients improve their lifestyle, but don't always take this advice themselves.

BURNOUT

Burnout is a term used very loosely to describe the consequences of job stress. It can mean anything from the need for a day off to becoming completely dysfunctional. In healthcare, there are many different causes for burnout including the obvious one of an overload of other people's trauma. Other causes are lack of control, sense of isolation, lack of community, lack of appreciation or lack of financial reward. I don't want to dwell on these as threats hanging over you; my intention is to raise your awareness and look at antidotes to burnout.

If you are a healthcare practitioner you have little control over outcomes. You can never predict accurately how much you can help anyone, however much a patient wants a promise of cure. You can make a good prognosis based on your previous experience but still have to live with not-knowing. The practice of mindfulness is the perfect answer to this, just being with the patient with no expectations.

You might feel quite isolated, either because you're practising on your own or because you have chosen a little-known therapy. The isolation and absence of like-minded community can mean that you don't get the peer support you need. If this is the case, you could increase your Internet connections.

Other stresses can be the lack of appreciation or positive feedback for your work from patients or from the general public. A patient who has had their problem relieved and is now feeling well often sees no point in returning to their practitioner and doesn't think to report the good news. You are often left wondering what happened, and maybe a quick courtesy phone call asking for feedback will boost your spirits. You can ask for the patient's feedback on the three separate areas of the consultation process, the treatment and the results. Often, simply doing this will result in a re-booking.

The symptoms of burnout are generally recognized as emotional exhaustion, depersonalization and lack of personal accomplishment. The burnt out practitioner finds it increasingly difficult to connect to and interact with their patients and colleagues. They generally become less responsive to all aspects of the work. Their body language and facial gestures demonstrate a reduced interest in other people and their problems. They disengage from colleagues and cut off from patients as individuals, seeing them as simply part of the daily routine. At the same time they lose any personal sense of achievement in the job.

Burnout can be expressed through changes in behaviour such as resistance to going to work, arriving late, postponing contact with patients or avoiding colleagues; changes in feelings such as graveyard humour or loss of sense of humour, loss of interest in everyday pleasures and feelings of failure, guilt, resentment or powerlessness; changes in thinking such as inability to concentrate, cynicism, or victim mentality; or changes in health such as disordered sleep, muscle tension, exhaustion and increased susceptibility to infection.

As part of their ethical framework, The British Association for Counselling and Psychotherapy (BACP) gives a clear statement about self-care that could be applicable to any other therapy:

> Attending to the practitioner's well-being is essential to sustaining good practice. Practitioners have a responsibility to themselves to ensure that their work does not become detrimental to their health or well-being by ensuring that the way that they undertake their

work is as safe as possible and that they seek appropriate professional support and services as the need arises. (p.9)

STRATEGIES FOR SELF-CARE

Following that depressing introduction on burnout, I have gathered together a list of strategies for self-care (see Box 12.1). The list is not complete, because there will always be new strategies to discover, and it is not in order of priority. I discuss all of them in more depth, and some of them have a chapter to themselves. The aim of all of them is to nourish and care for the physical body and/or the emotions and/or the spirit.

BOX 12.1 SOME STRATEGIES FOR SELF-CARE

- Taking care of your physical body
- Separation from the patient
- Relaxation, spoiling yourself and having fun
- Spending time with friends and loved ones
- Going to an alternative practitioner for yourself
- Contact with nature
- Getting support from colleagues
- Having compassion for yourself
- Balancing work with free time
- Self-awareness and self-monitoring
- Taming your inner judge and your inner justifier
- Having good boundaries (see Chapter 9)
- Mindfulness (see Chapter 5)
- Writing a self-reflective journal (see Chapter 13)

TAKING CARE OF YOUR PHYSICAL BODY

Some therapies are done while sitting in a chair or at a desk for many hours resulting in the practitioner not getting enough exercise. This happens, for example, in counselling, nutritional therapy or homeopathy. Body-work therapies and acupuncture often involve a lot of standing, which might be good for your legs, and bending over which is bad for your back. Therapies that involve massage or manipulation cause wear and tear to your hands and arms. All of us need exercise, and all of us need rest, and if you are out of balance with these two you will not function as well as you should. If you find yourself making excuses not to exercise, it probably needs to be set up as part of your routine. Fifteen minutes of walking a day is a very good starting point, and you can add one hour a week for an exercise class or sport.

Consider the other aspects of your physical health. Make a habit of eating well, with a commitment to good nutrition and monitoring your intake of food, drink, stimulants, alcohol and cigarettes. Aim to give yourself enough free time to wind down in the evenings so that you sleep well.

Do you go to an alternative practitioner for your own health or relaxation? It is an excellent experience to go to another practitioner in your field, and experience the therapy from the patient's viewpoint. It is equally good to try out different therapies that you did not know before. A good massage, a Reiki session or a shiatsu treatment are deeply relaxing as well as healing. Why not allow yourself a bit of luxury?

Contact with nature is very therapeutic. Yoga and Tai chi can be done outside or by a window where you can appreciate the different sorts of weather for what they are, and enjoy observing the turn of the seasons. Walking can be combined with mindfulness, the practice of keeping yourself totally present in the now, engaging with all of your senses while you walk. Cycling gives you fresh air, freedom and exercise as well as taking you to your destination. Being out in nature can be very refreshing on many levels: physical, emotional and spiritual – providing it is not the hayfever season.

Any form of exercise will help you to loosen up mind and body after a day in clinic. Many sports demand a lot of focus, keeping your attention on the activity and not allowing time in which you might ruminate on negative issues. Doing something that effectively turns your mind away from work can be very effective in reducing stress and the feelings of burnout.

Pet animals can be quietly demanding of their physical and friendship needs and have an excellent way of reminding you to take downtime from work. Spend time stroking your cat, taking your dog for a walk or talking to your chickens. (I know of several practitioners who keep chickens.)

RELAXATION, SPOILING YOURSELF AND HAVING FUN

Make the most of your time away from the intensity of your practice. You need to have downtime, when you are completely unavailable as a practitioner. You need time in which you can drop the responsibility of running a practice and have fun. Remember the simple delight of walking through dry, crunchy and colourful autumn leaves – or the magic of blowing iridescent bubbles into the sunshine (see Figure 12.1).

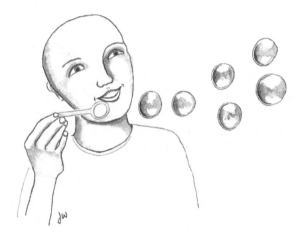

FIGURE 12.1: YOU'RE NEVER TOO OLD TO BLOW BUBBLES

Many people like to spoil themselves when they are on holiday, buying new clothes, going out for meals in the evening, or simply lying beside the pool getting a tan. These are big rewards that we give ourselves, after several months or a year at work. Are there any smaller rewards that you can give yourself on a more regular basis?

There are many activities that you can enjoy on your own, but they often increase in value if they are done with friends or loved ones. With people you are close to you can relax. With them you don't have to put on a professional front or look smart; you can simply be who you are. With friends, you can share food – or emotions – you can be spontaneous and you don't have to be consistently calm and focused. It is the opposite of your relationship with patients.

LAUGHTER

Laughter has been shown to have great healing benefits, on the physical, emotional, social and spiritual levels (see Box 12.2). It contributes to your quality of life. Laughter is the best antidote to burnout that I can think of. It stops you from taking life too seriously, and is at the polar opposite to vicarious trauma. It helps you relax and recharge, it decreases the stress hormones and it generally changes your perspective into a more positive one.

BOX 12.2 THE HEALING VALUES OF LAUGHTER

- Stress hormone levels decreased
- Well-being hormone levels increased
- Prevents heart disease
- Massage of abdominal organs
- Muscle relaxation
- Pain reduction
- Natural antidepressant
- Strengthens relationships
- Adds joy and zest to life

I'm sure that everyone could do with more laughter in their lives. The good news is that you don't have to wait for something funny to happen. You can try to smile more often and deliberately laugh more at amusing things. If you don't laugh easily, all that has happened is that your laughter reaction has gone to sleep and needs to be reawakened. If you're out of practice with laughter, you can build up your sense of humour again and become more spontaneous and less inhibited.

The brain cannot distinguish between spontaneous laughter and self-induced laughter, in the same way that it cannot distinguish between imagining something happening and the genuine experience. It appears that any form of laughter is healing, whether it is triggered by external stimulation or triggered by your own desire to laugh, and it can be with or without humour. If you are really out of practice with laughing, you may have to start with planned laughter rather than the spontaneous kind. That's okay! As an experiment, one day when you are alone in your home, try standing and laughing at nothing in particular for five minutes. Get your body used to the feeling and the sound of it, and get over your embarrassment. McGhee (1996) has researched the healing values of laughter for over 20 years. He writes about forcing yourself to laugh:

> This will seem artificial at first, but a funny thing happens after you force hearty laughter a few times. You start to feel its positive effects immediately, just as a smile somehow pulls you in the direction of feeling better. Laughter also helps focus your attention on the positive aspects of your life, which further boosts your morale and mood. (p.126)

Laughter can also act as a catalyst to release other emotions, for example suppressed grief can suddenly emerge when belly laughter turns to tears. McGhee (1996) writes, 'Even when laughter does not lead to crying, you can still feel a powerful cathartic release of pent-up tension, frustration, anger or anxiety' (p.127).

A lot can make you laugh, such as stand-up acts or comedy movies, your pet cat or dog, a piece of music, something you read, a witty remark, a light-hearted conversation or doing something silly yourself. The son of one of my colleagues searches the Internet for five- or ten-minute home movies. He wears headphones so that the first everyone else knows about it is hearing his infectious, chuckling laughter echoing from his bedroom.

SEPARATING FROM THE PATIENT

Emotions in a consultation can be contagious. Sometimes the patient's story can resonate with your own experiences, and thus reawaken your dormant emotions. If this happens, you might be tempted to stop listening to the patient, and focus on your inner world. At other times your brain's mirror neurons can directly copy the facial expressions of the patient and produce their emotions in you (see Chapter 9's section 'Emotional boundaries').

If you do find yourself carrying your patient's emotions, or you get headaches or other physical symptoms during or after the consultation, it might help to do a cleansing ritual after they have left. If you do a cleansing or clearing exercise it should be chosen by you as something that is effective for you. It is entirely personal, and the aim is to get rid of the previous patient's atmosphere in the room, as well as any foreign emotions that you copied from your patient and are still carrying.

You could open your clinic door and window, to allow some fresh air to flow through the room or light a candle or some incense. A deeper ritual is to take a shower, saying to yourself as the water flows over you, 'I am cleansing myself of this patient.' If you do not have time for a shower, careful hand-washing might suit you. A quick ritual is to brush yourself all over with your hands. Starting with your head, brush down your body, your arms and your legs, removing all traces of the patient. Using sound can make a very good clearing ritual. If you have a nice sounding bell or a ringing bowl, you can use it all the way round the perimeter of the clinic room. You could do five minutes of meditation to quieten your mind after any of these.

If you find you are regularly picking up the patient's issues, you might also need to do a protection ritual in the five or ten minutes before the patient arrives for their next appointment. Examples of protection exercises are to visualize yourself enclosed in a protective bubble, or sitting in behind a one-way mirror that you can see out of but the other person just sees a reflection of themselves. You can draw three circles in the air like hula hoops, one around your waist, another one front to back from floor to head, and the third one from side to side. A fun exercise is to put yourself into an imaginary sleeping bag and reaching down, grab hold of the imaginary zip and zip it slowly and carefully from your feet, past your knees, your waist, your chest, your neck and over your head. If this sounds claustrophobic, imagine plenty of space inside with a supply of fresh air.

GETTING SUPPORT

Support can come in many forms, from peers, spouses, friends, mentors, therapists and supervisors. The most immediate is what we might call coffee-break support, which is the five minute opportunity in which you tell a friend or colleague about your tough day and they sympathize. This acts as a brief relief of pressure, and is most welcome in the moment although it does not have a lasting effect. You might be able to do this with friends and family at home, but the ethics of confidentiality prevent you from sharing any details of your patients. However, they can be supportive in other ways, helping you make the most of your time off.

All the other forms of support contribute towards your overall self-development. The simplest, cheapest and often easiest is to meet with a critical friend for a session dedicated to helping each other. A critical friend is just that: someone who has your best interests at heart and feels warmly towards you, but is prepared to challenge you to think deeply and to encourage you to make changes to the way you work. A common arrangement is to divide the time between the two of you, so that each takes a turn at being critical friend for the other.

A peer group can be made up of people practising the same therapy, or different therapies. Meeting up as a support group is more than a coffee morning or a business meeting. It needs structure and a formally expressed aim or goal, such as: to support each other in our practices, treat each other with respect and appropriately challenge each other in order to develop and grow. A brief working agreement will clarify how you intend to work together, where you will meet, who would be chairperson (if necessary), how you will maintain confidentiality and how the time will be divided up.

The issue of allocating the time can be one of the most contentious in support groups. Imagine that you have a burning issue that you want to discuss with the group, but the practitioner who has the turn before you, decides to describe their issue with unnecessary minutiae and takes nearly double the amount of time that was allocated – which would leave you with just ten minutes to examine your issue. Whether this was intentional or bad timing makes no difference; your sense of irritation, frustration or injustice will not contribute towards the smooth running of the group or towards you working on your issue.

When I am facilitating small reflective groups, I start the session by asking everyone to give a 'headline' to describe what issues they want to explore in just one sentence. When we all know what everyone's issue is, we divide up the time appropriately and everyone knows how long they will get in the hot seat. As each participant has their turn, I encourage them to outline the story in the minimum of words and state clearly what help they want from the group. This allows them to have the larger percentage of their timeslot available for reflection and questioning from the rest of the group.

A peer group like this provides support and challenge for each member from the rest of the group. The whole group shares responsibility for supervising each other. The process of group work teaches everyone reflective questioning skills and increases everyone's understanding of the practitioner–patient relationship. The person in the hot seat gains insights into their particular issue as well as a deeper understanding of their patterns.

Another form of professional support is going regularly to an independent, fully qualified supervisor in order to explore your issues. This would be a confidential session, not reported back to those you work for. The advantage of working with someone who is trained as a supervisor is that they will be skilled in reflective questioning. They will encourage you to do much more than simply debrief, getting you to think deeply about what happened and learn from it. This exploratory process can be quite intense but contributes greatly towards your self-development and self-esteem.

Some supervisors just work with your cases, helping you to choose the best possible remedy or treatment plan and these have to be practitioners in the same therapy as you. But the supervisor who is interested in the relationship between you and your patient does not need to be from the same therapy. In my own experience, it can be quite stimulating to work with someone from a different discipline as their lack of understanding forces you to be really clear in your thoughts.

The supervisor who works with your practitioner–patient relationships and your practice generally, rather than your cases, does not need to be from the same therapy as you.

A practitioner came to see me for supervision, in order to work on her professional development plan. Her main issue was to build up her practice. She planned to complete her website, print up business cards with the same colours and font, and give a couple of small talks to the mothers at her grandson's nursery. She admitted that she felt very frightened about setting up a practice as she felt she was 'no good' at publicizing herself or giving talks. We talked about limiting beliefs (see Chapter 7) and how they could narrow her horizons and even cause her to sabotage her own success. I got her to write a list of things that she was 'good enough at' and as the list grew longer, she allowed herself a small smile of satisfaction. Then I asked her about the teaching and whether she really wanted to do it. There were other ways of advertising if she was not keen on it. She said that she loved working with children and although the mere thought of lecturing made her nervous, it seemed the best way to connect with the young mothers.

I picked up on the word lecturing and asked her for other words, both more formal and more informal. She suggested teaching, instructing and pontificating and began to laugh. Seeing her relax and lighten up, I suggested the words, enabling, assisting and facilitating. She was intrigued by these and I began to wonder out loud what it would be like to facilitate a gathering of people who would watch a demonstration and then discuss their experiences. She was thoughtful for a few minutes and then her ideas began to flow about working in a fun and interesting way.

If you share in a group practice or you are still at college, you might get support from tutors, college supervisors or managers. Their support will come in the form of feedback on your achievements and failures rather than reflective questioning. Feedback from them should be clear, owned, regular, balanced and specific (CORBS). Clear means transparent and easy to understand. Owned means that the person giving feedback takes responsibility for what they say rather than generalizing it ('I think' rather than 'people say'). Regular means that feedback should come every week, month or term. Balanced means giving an equal amount of negative feedback and positive feedback. Specific means explaining clearly what you mean, with detail if necessary.

Finally, what sort of support do you give yourself? My choice is that most of your self-reflections should include the questions, *What did I do well?* and *What didn't I do so well?* This creates balance in your feedback to yourself. Neff (2011) explains how our brains have a negativity bias as a survival mechanism:

> Our brains evolved to be highly sensitive to negative information so that the fight-or-flight response could be triggered quickly and easily in the brain's amygdala, meaning that our chances of taking action to ensure our survival would be maximized. Positive information isn't as crucial to immediate survival as it is to long-term survival…our brains give less time and attention to positive rather than to negative information. (pp.110–111)

Congratulating yourself can be done as a silent pat on the back, but it has more impact if it is said aloud to a colleague, critical friend or supervisor, or written down in the reflective journal. Putting the thought into concrete words gives it greater definition and power, either in writing where it can be reviewed, or saying it in front of a witness. Keeping a record of what is done well can consolidate good practice, boosting the self-confidence and providing much-needed support (see more about this in Chapter 1).

I have supervised many alternative practitioners who lack self-confidence because they cannot judge how good they are with their patients. They practise in isolation, and they miss the feedback from colleagues or managers. They could ask for feedback from their patients, but they find this difficult for fear it would be negative. They judge themselves according to cure rates rather than patient satisfaction. It does not occur to them to give balanced feedback to themselves, but once they start examining each consultation or treatment session and acknowledging what they did well, their confidence increases rapidly.

TAMING THE VOICES WITHIN

Everyone has an internal monologue, sometimes called intrapersonal communication, but more simply described as self-talk. This is a continuous stream of thoughts and feelings, a mixed commentary encompassing past, present and future, repeating itself and at times suddenly jumping topics. When something goes wrong or you have an experience that raises strong emotions for you, your self-talk focuses on that event. I have suggested in Chapter 3 that everyone carries an inner justifier and an inner judge, usually with one of them dominant.

Criticizing yourself as the judge or letting your inner justifier whine have the same effect in lowering your self-esteem. For many people there is a misunderstanding here. From childhood onwards we are used to people criticizing us as a way of motivating us, but actually it has the opposite effect. Criticism or self-criticism is demotivating and depressing and should be sandwiched between plenty of praise to be effective.

The first step towards quietening these inner voices is to increase your awareness that they are chattering again. Then you can start questioning them. Your mind is not the sum total of you. You can stand outside of your mind and notice what is going on inside it from the point of view of the unprejudiced observer, the leveller or the adult. Taking yourself into a state of meta-awareness where you are outside of your mind looking inward, is a moment of mindfulness. When you have meta-awareness, you can look dispassionately at your own thinking mind, and when it is being self-critical or self-justifying, ask, 'Is it true?' Writing in your reflective journal, list five or ten reasons why it is not true.

Routinely examining your self-talk as part of self-reflection can have a big impact on how you see yourself as a person as well as a practitioner. It can increase your self-knowledge and increase your self-confidence. Other ways of getting rid of your negative self-talk are working with the breath, Emotional Freedom Technique or Ho'oponopono from Hawaii.

To focus on your breath, take yourself into a meditative state, sitting still and connected to the floor through your feet or sitting bones if you are cross-legged. Focus softly on your breathing and relax. When you feel ready, with each in-breath invite in the strong, negative emotions you have noticed and fully acknowledge them. With the out-breath breathe them into the endless space around you. This is the space of kindness, mindfulness, compassion and common humanity. You might want to include a spiritual dimension to this as well. You can continue this for five to ten minutes.

Emotional Freedom Technique (EFT, sometimes known as tapping) can be done alone or with a practitioner. Specific points on the face and chest are tapped repeatedly by the fingertips while the patient speaks about any physical or psychological problems. It can be seen as related to neuro-linguistic programming, acupuncture and Thought Field therapy. Use it to free yourself from negative thoughts.

Ho'oponopono focuses healing energy through continuous repetition of the words, 'I'm sorry, please forgive me, thank you, I love you.' It is based on the ancient Hawaiian practice for the reconciliation of disputes which was done with the whole community. The premise is that we create the world around us through our thoughts – we are the sum total of all past thoughts – and we are all connected through divine energy, so each of us has to take responsibility for our own negative thought patterns. As we work to remove any negativity within us, the world around us is cleansed and healed. The process begins with the acknowledgement of our own negativity. The words are addressed to divinity (the higher self or the divine energy within us) beginning with an apology for the negative thought patterns that separate us from divine love and unity. We then ask for forgiveness, express love for divinity (which opens us up to receiving divine love) and give thanks to the divine for this opportunity to reconnect with all that is. This produces a state of mindfulness and of being in the now.

HAVE COMPASSION FOR YOURSELF

If you are regularly seeing patients, you will spend a lot of your day being compassionate towards other people. Learn to be compassionate towards yourself as well. Be as kind, considerate, caring, sympathetic, patient, concerned and gentle with yourself as you would be to them. You are not a different species, tougher and more immune to fatigue than other people. You are not a superhero who cures every case. You shouldn't have to be hard on yourself every time you achieve less than 100 per cent. You have chosen to practise your therapy because you believe in it and you like to help people. There is no doubt that you work hard.

The term 'drivers' comes from transactional analysis and refers to the driving forces that motivate people. These have been identified as: Be Strong, Hurry up, Try Harder, Be Perfect or Please People. Most people are motivated by two or three of these. They are internalized messages from our parents or carers about socially acceptable behaviour. Children try to conform to the behaviour their parents would like, in order to gain approval. However, following these drivers dogmatically can be restrictive or even dysfunctional. For example, the practitioner whose drivers are Be Strong and Please People will push themselves hard, taking on extra patients or teaching before admitting to stress. All of the drivers are open to self-criticism because you can never be strong enough/fast enough/perfect enough/try hard enough. Most of all, you can never please people enough – which is bad news for those of us in the caring or helping professions.

It can be interesting to do a drivers questionnaire to find out which are your main ones. (There are several questionnaires available on the Internet.) Once you know what to look for, you will see how many times your drivers dictate how you behave, and what attitudes and values you have. Remind yourself that drivers are not commandments set in stone. They're just something that you have inherited and you can soften them into something more rational. Drivers have the best interests of other people at heart (not you) and they appear to be just and fair to the whole community; but for you they can be hard task-masters with no consideration for your well-being. So be kind to yourself and tell your drivers that they are not always welcome.

When you make mistakes, you need to be honest about it with yourself, but you don't need to chastise yourself. Your inner judge is critical and would opt for a severe ruling. Your inner justifier is reaching for all sorts of excuses to explain why it's not your responsibility. Both of them are trying to protect you but they are not impartial and should be thanked and set aside. If you have built up trust writing in your journal or with your peer support group, critical friend or supervisor, then you can let go of the inner judge and inner justifier. As you investigate each experience you will gain understanding about what happened, why it happened and whether you need to make an action plan for the future. Many mistakes prove to be an excellent learning opportunity.

To avoid the voices of your inner judge and justifier, try to find some compassionate words that you would use for yourself. Say that you're doing okay and you don't need to drive yourself so hard. You can do this either in your mind while you're on the go or in your reflective journal. If you usually reflect with a critical friend, try getting them to listen while *you* show compassion to yourself. Whichever method you use, try to write up some notes afterwards in your journal, to remind you what you did and make suggestions for the next time you need to calm yourself.

Self-compassion, according to Neff (2011) has the three elements of loving-kindness towards yourself, awareness of belonging to common humanity and mindfulness. The first of these, giving yourself some loving-kindness, especially when things go wrong, might not be something you are used to doing. Loving-kindness is beyond simply comforting yourself with chocolate, cake or ice cream. It is changing your attitude so your inner voices are put on hold, and you do not feel the need to judge or justify. It is an acceptance of who you are, the way that your best friend accepts you with understanding, encouragement, patience and kindness. It says, 'There are some things that I do well, and some things I'm not so good at, and that's okay.' Neff (2011) writes:

> It's a great gift of self-kindness to have appreciation for ourselves, and to demonstrate our approval with sincere praise. We don't have to speak this praise aloud, making ourselves and others uncomfortable in the process. But we can quietly give ourselves the inner acknowledgement we deserve – and need. (p.272)

The second component of self-compassion is the awareness of belonging to common humanity. This means accepting that your experiences, no matter how painful, are part of the common human experience. You're not alone even when your experiences are suffering, grief, despair, anger or humiliation. Other people have been there. This might sound quite theoretical at first, until you include it in your self-talk. 'It's normal to feel like this, other people react like this, I'm not the only person to have done this, it feels painful right now but other people have experienced this and weathered the storm.'

The third aspect of self-compassion is mindfulness, which means being in the present moment, without dwelling on the past or trying to second-guess the future. Mindfulness is accepting that the only reality is this moment, now, and we can stop to appreciate the experience. The past has already gone and the future can only be imagined but never known, so you might as well trust the future will turn out well, and enjoy what you have now. 'I'm feeling tired as it's been a long day and the last case was difficult, but I don't feel I need to do anything right now, although it feels good to take my shoes off and stretch my feet. I have learnt a lot today, and I'd like to write it up in my journal, but just now I'm going to spend five minutes listening to my own breathing and relax.'

Sometimes you need to soothe yourself. To do this you should choose words that are calm, neutral, rational, balanced, blame-free, loving, and forgiving (like a caring Adult). It is often easier to generalize rather than be specific, so include words like *normally, usually, most of the time*, and so on. If you can, connect to something greater than yourself, such as your spiritual beliefs or by reminding yourself that other people have had similar experiences. I asked one of my study groups to reflect on this, first remembering a problem and then soothing themselves. When everyone had done this exercise, I told them that I did not want to know what the problem was, but I would like everyone to read out one sentence that soothed them. We had a wide variety of sentences such as: it's not the first time it's happened to me, I know I will be okay, usually I remember things, we are not the only couple to have arguments, it will be better in the morning, I don't have to think about it right now, normally I get very high grades, most of the time I know exactly what to do, every cloud has a silver lining, and the sun is shining today.

Another way to soothe yourself is to stroke your own skin as a mother might stroke her child. Once again the brain does not distinguish who is doing the stroking, whether it is someone who cares about you or you yourself. Either way you will release oxytocin and opiates which are the feel-good hormones.

DEVELOPING YOUR OWN STRATEGIES

In the early years of my practice I noticed that when my patients were not in front of me, I could completely forget what they looked like and what their symptoms were. I had to develop a way of writing up my notes that included a top sheet showing the main information, that I could glance through in the five minutes before the patient arrived and refresh my memory. More problematic were the times when patients rang up between appointments, and I wouldn't even recognize their name. 'I saw you last week' a patient would say and feeling very guilty I would reply, 'I'll just run and get your notes.' It was years later that I realized that this was an excellent protection device for me, so that I was unable to carry a patient between appointments, and arrived at each appointment with openness, a fresh curiosity, and a lack of expectation. My guilt and embarrassment aside, it became a very useful strategy for me.

As healthcare practitioners we all need strategies for letting go of the day's patients. I suggest that you should check regularly to see if you are caring enough for yourself. Do you remember to give yourself compassion, be kind to yourself when things go wrong and praise yourself to celebrate when things go well? Throughout the book I have written about various strategies that might help you keep a healthy balance between your practice and home life; there are lots more strategies out there that you can experiment with and adjust to suit yourself. Remember that you are a hard-working, giving person, and you deserve quality self-care.

REFLECTIVE EXAMPLE

What happened

A student came to see me for a homeopathic consultation yesterday. She is 20, and up until six months ago she was thoroughly enjoying being at university. She is clever and gets good exam results even though she doesn't study hard. She is also very pretty and has a busy social life; she indicates that she has had several boyfriends who were very attentive, although she is single now. Her parents are separated, and her home life seems to be rather unstable, but she's close to her brother.

Last summer, she decided to travel to South America with a group of friends, and then decided to do some further travelling on her own. The coach that she was travelling in went over the side of a cliff. No one was killed, but many of them were injured and help was a long time in coming. She herself was trapped, with her legs caught and it was some time before she was freed. Since then, she has lost her confidence and her cheerful, happy-go-lucky nature. She feels she has no one to talk to, and none of her friends at university understand her any more. She feels isolated and slightly detached from reality. When she went to a spa with some friends, she was not interested in gossiping with them, but felt really good spending time in the ice cold pool. She says that if homeopathy can't help her, she will try recreational drugs.

My feelings on hearing this story

She struck me from the beginning as interesting, because she was dressed very fashionably, almost frivolously, but her body language was restrained, her facial expressions reserved, and her tone of voice rather dull like someone who was depressed. I was shocked to hear of the coach crash, and felt great compassion when she spoke about her injuries and said none of her friends could understand her. I was upset by the consideration of recreational drugs, which felt rather like emotional blackmail: somehow forcing me to work harder so that I could 'save her' from hard drugs. I don't need that sort of pressure!

What I did well

I felt I was showing compassion, and I was aware of listening with great attention. I was focused on her, giving the occasional small prompts and my thoughts didn't wander, so I guess I was being Mindful. Looking at my case notes, I took a thorough case.

What I didn't do so well

I was concerned that I would show too much prejudice or become the admonishing Parent when she started talking about drugs, so I was concentrating on keeping a neutral face and missed the opportunity to give some gentle advice. I should have told her that although drugs might give temporary relief, they could entrench her in her detached state.

I did a good treatment agreement at the beginning of the session, but would have preferred to re-contract at the end. I could have negotiated how often she wanted see me and for how many appointments. I was too full of her story and I think I had picked up some of her dullness and detachment.

Where do I go from here?

Luckily she was my last client for the afternoon, so the first thing I did was to get out for a good walk, which refreshed me and revitalized my energy. Then I did my case analysis and sorted out a prescription for her.

I now need to decide about re-contracting with her. Do I send her a letter alongside the prescription, explaining how many sessions I will need to see her for? She might not read the letter, so it's probably better to phone her up, get her agreement, and send a letter to reiterate what we have agreed. I might also need to give her reminders before each appointment. As she is only a student, will there be a problem with money?

Issues to bring up at the next appointment

I need to clarify the re-contracting, so that she does come back regularly. This is a deep case and she has been mentally/emotionally unwell for six months. I would like to find out what other support she has: she told me she was close to her brother but I don't know what that means in practical terms.

My conclusion

I took a good case and I was compassionate. I feel that I have built up a good relationship with this girl and that she will return. I forgot to re-contract, but I can see that came from picking up some of her detachment. Next time she comes, I will sit a little further away from her, and give her slightly less eye contact. I will visualize myself sitting inside of a protective bubble. I will put a note on her file to remind me to check the re-contracting both at the beginning and at the end of the consultation.

EXERCISE: AUDIT YOUR SELF-CARE

First of all, decide what would be the ideal balance between your practice and your self-care. Be quite specific about this, considering different aspects of your work such as interviewing a new patient, doing the treatment or writing up your case notes. You can also consider the other aspects of self-care, such as food, exercise, time with friends, getting support and so on. Then choose some key questions that will help you monitor your balance between them, and keep records on a chart, or in your reflective journal or in your appointments diary. For example:

- Did I have a proper lunch break, away from my desk?

- Have I had some exercise today?

- Have I had time to communicate with a family member or friend, by phone, e-mail or text?

- Did I continue to think about clients at home or spend extra time in the clinic?

Do the audit for a month and then do an assessment in which you compare your ideal situation with reality. If there is a big gap between the two, start with small changes to improve the balance.

EXERCISE: DRAW YOUR SUPPORT NETWORK

Make a mind map with yourself in the centre. You can write your name, paste a photo or draw a picture of yourself. The rest of the mind map should be drawn like spokes to a wheel radiating from yourself at the hub. Each spoke should represent one aspect of your support, the whole finished mind map representing your support network. Spokes can have little branches coming off them. You can include things like your office, your massage table, your essential oils, getting exercise or growing your own vegetables. These are all on the physical realm. You might include emotional support provided by family, friends, pets, listening to music or going out into nature. You can include professional support, such as a critical friend, peer support groups, going to a supervisor or getting feedback from a manager. You could include intellectual support such as your computer, your books or going to seminars. You might want to include a spiritual dimension. You should *not* expect to get support from your patients.

To take this one step further, especially if you have already done the exercise, try to identify what manner of support you are receiving from each asset you have written down. For example, what do you get from your friends?

When you have finished the mind map, leave it for a day or so and then come back to it. Are there any areas in which you are missing support? If so, what can you do about it?

EXERCISE: LIFE IS SUPPOSED TO BE FUN

Writing your journal or doing a painting or drawing, try to identify what fun and laughter mean to you. How do you have your fun? What makes you laugh? Do you laugh on your own when there is no one around and do you feel comfortable laughing out loud along with other people? Do you have fun on your own or it is important to you to be with people? Are your pleasures simple like stroking your cat or are they complex like going out to the opera? Everyone is different and there are no right or wrong answers.

Make a list, a word cloud or a drawing of all the things that make you laugh and of all the things that are fun to do. Add in the things you would like to do that will be fun. The effort that you make in remembering them will bring them to the forefront of your mind, which will make you seek them out more often.

Chapter 13

THE SELF-REFLECTIVE JOURNAL

In my book on keeping a reflective journal, I describe self-reflection as:

> A process of observing what happens at work or at home, investigating it in order to understand it, and making suitable changes. It is an ongoing practice of refinement, made up of small steps. It can be done in a group, done one to one with a supervisor or critical friend, done online with a supervisor, or done alone. Doing it with someone else keeps the practitioner focused and on task, and challenges them to understand their issues at a deeper level. Reflecting alone requires more than just mulling it over while travelling home after a hard day at work. It needs discipline, serious inquiry and some way of storing the reflections for future reviews. Working with a self-reflective journal can fulfil all of these needs. (Wood 2012, p.9)

The aim of self-reflection is not to simply download your thoughts and feelings onto paper or screen; nor is it to judge or justify what has happened. The aim is to understand yourself better and introduce changes if necessary. It needs to be an honest investigation that is objective as far as possible. We could say that it needs the skills of case-taking, questioning yourself until you have fully understood the issue from an unprejudiced view point. It asks you to see the event or issue from the outside, as if you were watching a movie in order to review it.

The value of doing such an investigation is that you get to know new aspects of yourself and you can make positive changes to your attitudes, beliefs, values, thoughts or feelings. This will refine and improve the way you work and benefit your patients, your practice and your profession. I suggest there are many different ways of doing self-reflection and it is up to you to choose what suits you. There are numerous examples throughout this book of different ways to reflect.

You can write about anything at all. Reflections can be about your professional life, home life or studies. They can be used to explore the past such as an analysis of what has gone well or an investigation into what hasn't gone well. They can also be used to plan the future using methods like brainstorming, goal setting or visualization. Some books recommend that you should only reflect on 'critical incidents' but if this is all you use reflection for, you are limiting its possibilities.

In the same way, I would not want to limit journal entries to any particular format. I have demonstrated several different styles in reflective examples throughout the book, but these are all left-brained, logical and written. Some people prefer to do an art journal or a scrapbook journal and these, or any other combination of words and pictures, are equally valid.

A practitioner once explained to me why she didn't keep a journal herself. 'Why would I want to keep a record of all the times I criticize myself?' Why indeed? She found she got much more support from her monthly supervision group, and if she had an urgent problem she could book one-to-one supervision with the group facilitator. She hadn't thought of the journal in terms of supporting herself. I suggest that we need both external support from others, and internal support from ourselves.

SOME GUIDELINES FOR SELF-REFLECTION

BOX 13.1 GUIDELINES FOR SELF-REFLECTION

- Be honest about the objective story.
- Acknowledge your feelings about what happened.
- Express yourself openly.
- Investigate from the position of the unprejudiced observer.
- Have compassion for the patient and for yourself.
- Write down what you have learned.
- Create an action plan.
- Re-read or revisit old issues to observe change.

I am offering some guidelines for self-reflection, but it is not a finite list; some things might not be relevant and you might want to add to it (see Box 13.1). If you're writing about something that has happened, try as far as possible to differentiate between what actually happened and how you feel (or felt) about it. These two tend to get twisted up together and your feelings will colour the story. It might feel difficult at first but you will soon become better at identifying the objective account and acknowledging and expressing your subjective feelings. You might find your feelings change, the further away you get from the incident or dilemma. That's okay, just acknowledge your changing feelings. You might want to name your feelings, but if you're using a creative method such as painting, to investigate your issue then your feelings could be expressed through colour and shape without being named.

Identifying the difference between the subjective and the objective could be a reflection in itself but frequently you will want to go onto the next stage, which is investigation. This might be a logical analysis, maybe warranting research through books; but it could also be doing something creative to allow your subconscious to reveal itself. The journal is the best possible place to write down what you have learnt. Take note if your inner judge or your inner justifier step onto the stage. They too can be investigated through questions like, 'Is this true?' or 'Where does this come from? Who said this to me?' Finally, decide whether you need to create an action plan. This won't be necessary every time and in some cases I have found the shift in understanding is so profound that the attitude changes from the inside; and an action plan would limit possibilities.

If you're writing about something that might happen or you want to happen in the future, then use your journal to raise your emotional level. It is important to acknowledge any feelings of doubt or negativity when goal setting, but having done so, I suggest you put them to one side and focus on raising your positive energy. Negativity will hold you back from what you want to achieve, so spend some time imagining how good it will feel when you have reached your goal. You could write a word cloud using only positive words. (A word cloud is simply a cluster of random words within a cloud like shape.) You could do a drawing or painting of what it would feel like when you get there.

However deep you dig into your thoughts and feelings when writing your journal, try to include some compassion in the conclusion.

This could be for the other people you are writing about and/or for yourself. Self-compassion has three facets or stages according to Neff (2011) that flow from yourself and how you are feeling right now, to the wider human experience and back to yourself with a spirit of kindness and understanding. I call this soothing yourself, a process of gently talking to yourself in a calming and reassuring way like, 'These things happen, other people have been here, it's okay, I can learn from this, I deserve to feel good, all is well.'

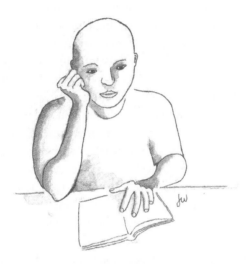

FIGURE 13.1: LEARN EVEN MORE ABOUT YOURSELF
THROUGH RE-READING YOUR JOURNAL

One of the real advantages of keeping a self-reflective journal is that of re-reading previous entries. You will start to see patterns emerging of experiences repeating themselves; and you will learn even more about yourself. You will also see old issues that you have completely left behind because they are no longer a problem and you might feel slightly surprised that they were such a big deal at the time. You might want to add a postscript to a previous entry to give an update, or do a new reflection on what you have discovered through re-reading old reflections (see Figure 13.1).

STRUCTURED REFLECTION OR GO WITH THE FLOW

Time willing, everything can be explored through self-reflection. For example, a situation arises between yourself and a colleague.

Things were said – or not said – that have left you feeling upset, angry or frustrated. You can get coffee-break support from another colleague or you could take it to a peer group or supervisor to try and understand what happened at a deeper level – or you could use your journal. Choosing a journal style that suits you (see below), you could begin to gently question yourself in order to reveal what happened and how you feel about it. You could explore it to uncover any hidden thoughts, attitudes, values or assumptions.

If we concentrate on the aim of self-reflection, which is to understand yourself better for the benefit of you, your patient and your practice, then it shouldn't matter how it is done. There are many different techniques available, and as long as the technique you use enables you to dig deep, then choose the one that suits you. If you are having difficulties with self-reflection, it might be because you're trying to work in a style that doesn't suit you.

In the early part of the last century it was presumed that everyone learned through listening to the teacher and then practising it for themselves. More recently it has become generally accepted that everyone has their own preferred learning style. These are generally grouped into fact-finding, analysing or working with one of the senses such as visual, aural, tactile or oral learning styles – or a mixture of a couple of them. You might find that you learn better on your own or you may prefer to learn in a group. You could need a lot of stimulation to learn or you might prefer plenty of time, peace and quiet.

It is the same with the self-reflective journal. If your intention is to understand yourself and your issues, it can be done equally well with the logical, analytical left brain or with the intuitive, perceptive right brain – or both. Students are often taught that they should use a reflective framework so as to analyse the issue efficiently, but for some people creative expression takes them much deeper. Finding a reflective style that suits you might really open up your reflections – or you might find that using one technique all the time makes you bored, complacent or superficial. The brain enjoys a challenge, so you might prefer to have several different reflective techniques to swap between.

REFLECTIVE FRAMEWORKS AND MODELS

Structured reflective techniques, such as reflective cycles, take you step-by-step through a series of logical questions. An example is the cycle by Gibbs (1988). It has six different stages, starting with the objective question 'What happened?' This is followed by 'What were you thinking and feeling?' This question allows you to be totally subjective and explore your reactions to what happened. The third question asks you to weigh up what you did well and what you didn't do so well. 'What was good and bad about the experience?' It then asks you to analyse what happened with the questions, 'What sense can you make of the situation?' and 'What else could you have done?' Finally you are asked, 'If the situation arose again, what would you do?' This last question is perhaps not so relevant for people in the helping professions where every situation is different from the previous, but we can loosely translate the last question as: 'What do you need to do now?' Keeping your reflections within a framework like this provides trigger questions that enable you to cover several different aspects that you might otherwise have missed. An example of the Gibbs (1988) reflective cycle is the reflection at the end of Chapter 12.

A different framework is Borton's (1970) developmental model, which has three simple questions: 'What? So what? Now what?' The first question gets you to identify what happened or what the issue is about. The second question asks about the consequences and the third one is the action plan. Because this cycle is quite general, it is flexible. Each question can have numerous answers, and the topic could be an incident from the past, a current dilemma or a decision for the future. An example of Borton's (1970) developmental model is the reflection at the end of Chapter 4.

I used this reflective framework to consider a patient that I had been seeing for nearly a year:

What?
For the first six months she made very good progress with an improvement in both her bowel symptoms and her self-confidence among strangers. She became less irritable with her partner and noticeably woke up in the mornings in a better mood. Then she missed an appointment and had to postpone the next one. The symptoms all began to return and she sent me a text asking if I could repeat the prescription without seeing her.

So what?
I agreed reluctantly, knowing that it would be more professional to see her and take a full case, but feeling sympathetic towards her anxiety about her

re-emerging symptoms. I didn't hear from her for another two months when she asked for another prescription. When I asked her to come in for a check-up, she said the symptoms were the same as before and she didn't have the time or money for an appointment.

So what?
It was now several months since I had seen her face-to-face, and I needed to do a full case-taking again. I would be unprofessional to prescribe after such a long time of not seeing her.

So what?
I felt uncomfortable with the tone of her text messages. I find it hard to accept that she did not have time or money for an appointment. I did not like the way she implied this was my responsibility, as if my fees were an unfair indulgence on my part.

So what?
Maybe this was my fault for sending her the first distance prescription. Maybe I set up her expectations that I would continue to do this.

Now what?
Although it feels unethical to abandon a patient, it is also unethical to prescribe without seeing her. I will send her my terms and conditions again to remind her of our working agreement.

A different type of structured framework, is the SWOT chart (credited to Albert Humphrey 1960s–70s in Stanford University). This invites you to list your strengths, weaknesses, opportunities and threats, which are written in a box divided into four equal parts. I have described this elsewhere (Wood 2012) as 'brainstorming with structure'. It can be completed in any order. I suggest that you start the process with a sentence expressing a goal or a question, and then use the four different headings to examine it from different angles. Be honest about your weaknesses but don't dwell on them, and celebrate and feel proud of your strengths. Examine opportunities on every level, physical, mental or emotional. The threats are the things that might go against you and make it difficult for you to achieve your goal.

A practitioner asked me for some supervision because he was uncertain whether to join a new clinic, so we worked with the SWOT chart. His strengths were that he could work well in a team and he was qualified in a couple of different therapies. His weakness was that he found it difficult to finish on time and someone else might have booked the room after him. The opportunities were many: he would have more patients referred to him, he would get to know other practitioners, he would be put on the clinic website and the clinic was close enough to bicycle there. The threat was that the clinic fees were expensive and he would have to pay even if he didn't have any bookings.

Some reflective techniques are less structured than these frameworks, but nonetheless very helpful in triggering new ideas and insights. One of these is the technique that I call 'fork in the road'. This is a way of reflecting on a decision that was made in the past or a decision that needs to be made for the future. Consider a situation where everything was going smoothly until you reach a fork in the road where you have to make a decision. You make the choice as wisely as you can, but you can't help thinking what would have happened if you had chosen the other route. Taking into consideration what you know and understand about the issues involved, ask yourself the question, 'What if…?' You can use this to explore what might have happened if you'd taken the other fork in the road or the opposite decision. You might have to ask 'what if' several times.

CREATIVE SELF-REFLECTION

The structured reflective cycles always start with an objective description of what happened, and then progress to analysing your feelings. Creative reflection starts directly with the subjective, expressing emotions through the use of creative media such as painting, collage or music, and re-examining it later for further insights. Afterwards a few notes are recorded in the reflective journal about the creative process and any thoughts that arise from the following questions: 'What have I learned from this?' and 'What should I do now?' You could also write a short summary of the objective story.

Artwork can be done through painting, drawing, collage, modelling materials and any other media. Before you start, take a few minutes to immerse yourself in the emotions surrounding your issue. Try to remember what it felt like to be with that patient or colleague or imagine what it will feel like when you get that job. If this isn't helpful for you, then sit for a few minutes in quiet meditation, encouraging your mind to slow down and arrive in the now. Then quietly gather together the materials you might need, such as drawing paper, glue, felt tip pens or paints. Allow yourself to draw or paint intuitively and expansively, immerse yourself in the creativity and don't think about the end result. Then leave it alone without looking at it for a few hours or a few days. When you return to it you can start to analyse it from a more intellectual mindset.

When you come back to your artwork look at it with fresh eyes and from the position of the Adult, leveller or unprejudiced observer, and review what you have done. What can you learn from the colours you chose, the textures, the gaps of white paper showing through, the exaggerations of line or shape, or the energy expressed? What is your unconscious mind telling you? What new thoughts are being triggered?

As part of a workshop on self-reflective journaling, I invited the participants to flick through a pile of magazines and newspapers and cut out any picture or headline that took their fancy within the title of 'Me and My Family'. They were to interpret this title in any way they wanted. The first thing I noticed was the intense, absorbed atmosphere as the participants searched almost blindly for pictures that resonated. If they had done this exercise at home, they might have taken time to decide what pictures they wanted and searched for them. In the workshop they had to keep an open mind and take the pictures that felt right. When they had chosen enough pictures they were asked to make a montage.

We went on to an entirely different exercise before returning to the montage, when I asked them to look at it with their thinking mind and make notes. Then I asked them to work in pairs, and give some feedback on what they observed about each other's montage. I overheard warm and constructive feedback, such as, 'I notice there is a lot of grey in your pictures, and I was wondering if this is your favourite colour because to me, grey symbolizes…'; 'I like the way that the red bird is at the centre of the picture. It gives me a sense of liveliness and energy.'; 'I notice that you have chosen a very symmetrical layout and I'd like to ask if your home life is very organized or not?'

Another way of reflecting creatively is to explore symbolism. Choose a story, myth or fairytale, or a character out of one of these to represent your issue. A supervisee once said to me, very cautiously, 'I don't think I like my patient very much.' I asked whether the patient reminded her of anyone, expecting to be told about a person from her past. She was quiet and thoughtful for a long time and eventually said, 'I can't think of anyone directly. I don't usually meet that sort of person... She's a bit like the White Queen in Alice in Wonderland, who's always screaming before she gets hurt... A fussy hypochondriac.' The practitioner introduced this symbol, with no disrespect to the patient, and I decided to take it further. I could understand the patient might be a hypochondriac like the White Queen – but I thought we could explore whether this patient had any other Queen-like characteristics, such as haughtiness or bossiness. Another example of using symbolism is the reflection at the end of Chapter 2.

Other ways of self-reflecting with symbolism are to transfer the characteristics of your patient, your colleague or yourself into another kingdom in terms of animals, plants or minerals. You might choose to look at your patient as an animal. Again, no disrespect is intended. If your patient is extroverted, friendly, sexual, enthusiastic and a little bit scatty, you may choose to represent her as a young lioness or a dolphin. If you enjoy her company you might choose another of the big cats or large sea creature for yourself; but if you choose a small animal for yourself it might reveal you are a bit nervous or in awe of her. If you choose something opposite in character for yourself, this could reveal aspects of yourself or the patient that you hadn't been aware of before. This method of self-reflection won't be useful if you're very literal minded.

Sometimes you have to follow your intuition or inner knowing in order to unravel an issue in your journal, especially if it concerns another person. This might sound unscientific to the logical thinker, but consider how much information you unconsciously pick up through observing the body language of another person. If you can tap into that hidden store of information you might understand the other person better and through doing this get to know new aspects of yourself. As with all the other techniques in this chapter, this should be done after the patient has left, not in front of them.

Place two chairs opposite each other and designate one for yourself and one for the other person. If you don't have two chairs, you could make a drawing of this or just do it in your imagination. Tell the story from your own point of view, sitting in your chair.

Stand up and have a stretch when you have finished your point of view and then sit in the other chair, literally or metaphorically. Spend a few minutes remembering the other person, and then copy their body language as well as you can remember it and mime their facial expression or hand gestures as a way of getting under their skin. Then tell the story from their point of view. Do it with compassion and gentleness. You'll be surprised how much you know about their opinions even though you have reached it through intuition.

I did this exercise with a student who was feeling very guilty about taking a clinic case when she was unwell. She had had a streaming cold and her concentration was impaired, which in turn made her question what her patient thought of her. She was sure he thought she was unprofessional and was probably very irritated with her. However, after sitting in the patient's chair, she realized with amazement that the patient was so full of his own story and his own concerns that he hadn't noticed her condition at all. He trusted her from previous consultations and was not judging her efficiency. As the student realized this it was as if a weight had fallen off her shoulders. She started to laugh about how she had put herself at the centre of the consultation after the event, whereas at the time the patient had been there.

PRACTISE SELF-COMPASSION

Your self-reflective journal should nourish you and help you to grow in wisdom and compassion. Your inner judge and inner justifier will want to be heard but they will tend to keep you in the same place without learning anything new. Try not to listen to them (they are not who you are) and write at the front of the journal your decision to be kind to yourself.

BOX 13.2 PRACTISE SELF-COMPASSION

- Write about the good as well as the bad.
- Praise yourself for what you did well.
- Soothe yourself when things go wrong.
- Appreciate everything.

I suggest that you should consciously use your journal to acknowledge and praise yourself for what you do well. If you find this difficult then it is probably because you're very self-critical and you're out of practice of being kind to yourself. It's time to start now. If you feel embarrassed or awkward doing it, perhaps because you were told as a child not to boast, then try having some fun with it. You could give yourself a gold star or a smiley face, write your good points in a larger font or more cheerful colour than in writing about your failures. An example is the reflection at the end of Chapter 1.

If you do have failures, soothe yourself to take the sting out of it. Soothing yourself is not the same as self-justification. It is calming yourself into a more neutral place that is neither critical nor defensive. You might write in your journal something like: 'That's interesting, I never knew that about myself. It feels a bit strange seeing myself in that light, but other people have the same vulnerabilities, I'm not the only one. It was really tough for me and I can see why I got frustrated but it's not the end of the world. It's understandable that I feel a bit raw at the moment, so I think I'll just relax this evening and follow through my action plan tomorrow morning.'

Neff (2011) writes 'self-kindness allows us to see ourselves as valuable human beings who are worthy of care' (p.49). She goes on to say:

> When we experience warm and tender feelings towards ourselves, we are altering our bodies as well as our minds. Rather than feeling worried and anxious, we feel calm, content, trusting, and secure. Self-kindness allows us to feel safe as we respond to painful experiences, so that we are no longer operating from a place of fear – and once we let go of insecurity we can pursue our dreams with the confidence needed to actually achieve them. (p.49)

APPRECIATION AND GRATITUDE

Another way of using your journal to nourish yourself is to express gratitude and appreciation. These two are very similar and both demonstrate pleasure in the way things are turning out. Gratitude has more of an element of thankfulness (e.g., to the self, to other people, to the planet, to the universe, to spirit) while appreciation has more delight or love. Gratitude says: 'Thank you for something that you have just done or will do' while appreciation says: 'Everything is wonderful!' or 'You are amazing.' It doesn't matter which way you express it, but if you can take time every day to feel pleasure in the good things in life, or simply the good things in your practice, you will significantly raise your mood and your energy.

Youngson (2012) describes the self-healing that occurs when you consciously use these positive emotions:

> When you exercise the positive emotions of gratitude, appreciation, compassion and loving kindness you cause structural changes to occur in your brain. It's not called 'the practice of compassion' for nothing. The centres associated with positive emotions and pro-social behaviours actually grow bigger, create more connections, and increase their blood supply.
>
> Over time you will achieve greater resilience, equanimity, happiness and contentment. Everyday irritations will lose their power to trigger negative emotions. You will become much less prone to disorders of anxiety and depression.
>
> These changes are also associated with significant improvements in physical health including lowered blood pressure, enhanced immune function, and reduced risk of heart disease. (p.97)

Use your journal as a place to appreciate the good things in life. Try writing a list of what has gone well every evening for a couple of weeks. Include even the smallest things, such as the bus arriving just after you got to the stop, the shopkeeper smiled at you, your patient arrived on time, you arrived on time, you did a very good treatment, you saw some flowers in someone's window, your partner cooked for you or you found the time to do half an hour's exercise. You can write about these as a list in a strictly factual way or you can turn them into a narrative story. You can express them emotionally through the words of loving kindness or you can write them as a poem. You can have fun representing them artistically.

You can deliberately increase the feel-good factor by injecting a lot of enthusiasm into the words you have chosen. This can give you a real boost, making you feel great and very positive about your work. This could be something like, 'I woke up to sunshine this morning, I love waking up to sunshine, I feel really good about my practice, I had such a lovely patient this morning, she had done everything I recommended and I feel great about that, she is a real joy to work with. Because the sunshine was so warm and bright this morning, I decided I would like to fit in a walk sometime in the day, and my first phone call today was from patient X who wanted to postpone her appointment. So there was free time for my walk, which was amazing!'

If you receive any appreciation or gratitude from others, accept it and keep it, even if you don't think you have earned it. Allow others to express their opinion if they feel you have helped them. This is no time to modestly shrug your shoulders and bypass praise from others. You need to record it in your journal to boost yourself on a bad day. It can come from patients, peers, managers, tutors or supervisors. If someone expresses verbal appreciation for your treatments, jot it down and put it into your self-reflective journal. Keep an appreciative e-mails folder or better still, copy and paste them into your journal where you can re-read them. If your journal is of the paper kind, you can print out e-mails to paste into the journal, along with notes or cards from people who appreciate your work.

CHOOSE WHO YOU WANT TO BE

Journals and personal diaries go in and out of fashion, and if you're not used to writing about yourself it might appear to be an unnecessary chore that takes up your spare time. But the reflective journal is worth the effort as you get to know yourself better. It gives you the opportunity to shed some of the unnecessary beliefs and attitudes that you've been carrying since childhood. You will be able to choose who you really want to be as a person and as a practitioner. Using self-reflection, you can blame yourself less, praise yourself more and become more compassionate towards yourself.

REFLECTIVE EXAMPLE

My patient numbers have gone down over the last few months. It might be quite simply that the recession is affecting all alternative therapies – which is what I've been saying to myself. But the other thing is that I've been turning my energies away from my practice, allowing it to tick-over without giving it much love and attention. A lot has been going on and I've been busy, and to some extent I appreciated having fewer patients around while my dad was ill. He's better now and it's time to turn my attention back to my practice.

What I would like to do is a sort of spring cleaning or space clearing of my whole practice! But first of all I need to decide what that would entail and whether it is realistic in terms of time and money.

What I'm good at

- making my patient feel safe and comfortable
- making a practical working agreement with the patient
- being mindful throughout the session
- finding appropriate questions and listening attentively to the patient
- noticing and responding appropriately to the patient's tone of voice, body language and facial expressions
- planning and negotiating with the patient at the end of the session.

What I'm not so good at

- booking in the next appointment for my patient
- advertising, social networking and generally updating my website
- sending an invoice for missed appointments.

It looks as if I have excellent people skills, but I'm not good at the office skills of booking in, charging and advertising. To be honest I find this sort of stuff boring, so I do tend to avoid doing it and haven't bothered to update my knowledge. I'm a bit annoyed with myself because I should have realized this earlier – office stuff has always been my weakness – no wonder my practice is diminishing.

Now wait a minute! That last sentence was the voice of my inner judge telling me off. I don't want to listen to it: I've been very busy for the last three months and it was very stressful when my dad was ill. I've given all my available time to my loyal, long-term patients. Hmm, this sounds like my inner justifier is having a go now.

Soothing myself

I am pleased that I spent time with my long-term patients when dad was ill. I'm sorry I dropped a lot of the office work. But it was a good strategy. It reduced the amount of stress I was under. Most people would do the same. I wouldn't have helped anyone if I had become burnt out. Now I've got more time, I can pick it up again. More than that, I'm planning to reassess and refresh how I manage the administration. This feels like a good time to put energy into my practice and make a fresh start. It could be fun!

What I plan to do

1. I will do an audit starting next week on my end-of-session administrative work with my patients. I will keep it in the back of my

diary and run it for a month. It will be a tick-chart to monitor whether I take the fees and book in the next appointment with each patient. I will make sure that patients who miss appointments are also recorded on this chart. I hope that putting energy into making the chart and keeping it up to date will act as a reminder as well as a research tool. It will measure whether I am as lax as I think I am about booking in or sending invoices. Making a tick-chart does not seem too demanding or boring. It is realistic in terms of my time and money criteria.

2. I will refresh and update my website. This means reading through everything meticulously and editing what I have written. Then I need to decide whether I like the layout and whether it can be changed easily with new photos, or whether it would be better to scrap it and start again. In terms of my time and money criteria, this is a project that will run over several weeks, and might prove quite expensive if I decide to go for a new website. I will need to assess what needs changing and investigate prices. On the other hand it will be easy to get new photos taken and I can ask my critical friend to proofread the new text. More importantly, even as I'm writing about it now, I can feel a sense of excitement and vitality, so the energy is already beginning to return. This shows me that I am definitely on the right track!

EXERCISE: APPRECIATE YOURSELF

Spend ten minutes every evening writing a list of things that you did well during the day, even if it includes such mundane things as filing the patient notes or remembering to make that phone call. Anything positive that you tell yourself will be a boost to your confidence. Write at least six of these acknowledgements of small achievements. Then write down at least ten things that you appreciated about your day. These could be as simple as the sun was shining, someone smiled at you at the bus stop, a patient followed your instructions, someone made a referral to you, a patient reported that they felt better after your last treatment or you were able to explain yourself clearly on the phone.

EXERCISE: BE CREATIVE

Think about the healing modalities that you practise and decide how they benefit *you*. You might consider advantages like these: being able to help patients, meeting interesting people, the mental challenge of finding a good prescription, feeling their energy or Chi, boosting your own vital energies, and so on. Find as many reasons as possible why you have become – and remain – an alternative practitioner, and put them into your journal as either a mind map, a collage or a drawing/painting. If you're doing a mind map it should have yourself at the centre, with radiating lines leading to all of the different aspects, rather like the spikes that surround a child's drawing of the sun.

EXERCISE: INVESTIGATE REFLECTIVE FRAMEWORKS

There are many different reflective frameworks available. I have given you a few examples, but there are many more. You can find several in my book, *Transformation through Journal Writing* (Wood 2012) or you can do an Internet search. When you have investigated several, test out one or two. Choose a simple subject such as something that surprised you during the Christmas holidays, and put it through your chosen reflective framework. See what you can learn from doing this. Did the framework suit you? If it irritated you, consider why. Did you find yourself amending it? If it did suit you, would you use it again?

REFERENCES

British Association for Counselling and Psychotherapy (BACP) Lutterworth: BACP. Available at www.itsgoodtotalk.org.uk/assets/docs/BACP-Ethical-Framework-for-Good-Practice-in-Counselling-and-Psychotherapy_1360076878.pdf British Association for Counselling and Psychotherapy, accessed on 3 April 2014.

Berne, E. (1961) *Transactional Analysis in Psychotherapy*. New York: Grove Press Inc.

Bond, T. (1993) *Standards and Ethics for Counselling in Action*. London: Sage Publications.

Borton, T. (1970) *Reach, Teach and Touch*. London: McGraw Hill.

Brown, K.W. and Ryan, R.M. (2003) 'The benefits of being present: Mindfulness and its role in psychological well-being.' *Journal of Personality and Social Psychology 84*, 4, 822–848.

Falkner, D. (2013) 'Back to the source, the power of objective observation.' *The Homeopath 32*, 1, 13–17.

Fox, S. (2008) *Relating to Clients: The Therapeutic Relationship for Complementary Therapists*. London: Jessica Kingsley Publishers.

Gibbs, G. (1988) *Learning by Doing: A Guide to Teaching and Learning Methods*. Oxford: Further Educational Unit, Oxford Polytechnic.

Gilbert, P. (2009) *The Compassionate Mind*. London: Constable & Robinson.

Hahnemann, S. translation by J. Künzli, A. Naude and P. Pendleton (1986) *Organon of Medicine*. London: Victor Gollancz. (Original published in 1810.)

Kaplan, B. (2001) *The Homeopathic Conversation: The Art of Taking the Case*. London: Natural Medicine Press.

Karpman, S. (1968) 'Fairy tales and script drama analysis.' *Transactional Analysis Bulletin 7*, 26, 39–43.

Katie, B. (Copyright Byron Katie Mitchell 2002) *Loving What Is: Four Questions That Can Change Your Life*. New York: Random House.

Lapworth, P. and Stills, C. (2011) *An Introduction to Transactional Analysis*. London: Sage Publications.

Lipton, B. (2005) *The Biology of Belief: Unleashing the Power of Consciousness, Matter and Miracles*. London: Hay House.

Losier, M. (2007) *Law of Attraction: Getting More of What You Want and Less of What You Don't*. London: Hodder & Stoughton.

Maslow, A.H. (1943) 'A theory of human motivation.' *Psychological Review 50*, 4, 370–396.

McGhee, P.E. (1996) *Health, Healing and the Amuse System: Humour as Survival Training*. Iowa: Kendall/Hunt Publishing.

Neff, K. (2011) *Self Compassion: Stop Beating Yourself Up and Leave Insecurity Behind*. New York: William Morris.

Neighbour, R. (2005) *The Inner Consultation: How to Develop an Effective and Intuitive Consulting Style.* Abingdon: Radcliffe Publishing.

Pease, A. and Pease, B. (2004) *The Definitive Book of Body Language: How to Read Others' Attitudes by their Gestures.* London: Orion Books Ltd.

Rogers, C. (1961) *On Becoming a Person.* Boston: Houghton Mifflin.

Rothschild, B. (2006) *Help for the Helper. A Psychophysiology of Compassion Fatigue and Vicarious Trauma.* New York, London: W.W. Norton.

Santorelli, S. (1999) *Heal Thy Self: Lessons on Mindfulness in Medicine.* New York: Three Rivers Press.

Schuck, C. and Wood, J. (Winter 2007) 'Creating boundaries in the consulting room.' *Society of Homeopaths Newsletter.*

Seligman, M.E.P. (2011) *Flourish, a New Understanding of Happiness and Well-Being – And How to Achieve Them.* London: Nicholas Brealey Publishing.

Silverman, J., Kurtz, S. and Draper, J. (2005) *Skills for Communicating with Patients.* Oxford: Radcliffe Publishing.

Townsend, I. (2011) *More Than Just A Drop in The Ocean? Finding the Person-Centered Approach in Homeopathy.* Paper presented at 25th Anniversary Meeting of the Association for the Development of the Person-Centered Approach, University of Loyola, Chicago, IL, July 27–31, 2011. Unpublished mono available from ian. townsend@yahoo.co.uk

Wood, J. (2012) *Transformation through Journal Writing: The Art of Self-Reflection for the Helping Professions.* London: Jessica Kingsley Publishers.

Youngson, R. (2012) *Time to Care: How to Love Your Patients and Your Job.* New Zealand: Rebelheart Publishers.

INDEX

TRANSFORMATION THROUGH JOURNAL WRITING
The Art of Self-Reflection for the Helping Professions
Jane Wood

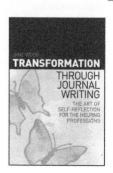

Paperback: £15.99 / $24.95

ISBN: 978 1 84905 347 1

240 pages

Transformation through Journal Writing is a grounded guide to self-reflection through journaling for those in the helping professions. Journals are shown to be an effective method of self-care and self-development.

Full of inspiring and original ideas, this book provides everything you need to know about developing and advancing journaling skills. It covers a range of different styles, from the logical and structured use of templates, frameworks and models, to the creative and organic process of art journaling. Each technique and its transformative potential are clearly explained, and readers are encouraged to start writing through expertly crafted exercises and journal examples. It is a flexible resource that will inspire readers to start a reflective journal for the first time or to try out new techniques and methodologies.

A comprehensive handbook to self-reflective journaling, this book will be of interest to everyone in the health professions including complementary and alternative practitioners, supervisors, counsellors, psychotherapists, and art, music and drama therapists.

Contents: Preface. 1. Introducing the Reflective Journal. 2. Getting Started. 3. Narrative Journal. 4. Essential Tools for Reflective Journals. 5. Advanced Tools and Techniques. 6. Creative and Art Journals. 7. Reflective Frameworks and Models. 8. Visualisation. 9. Reflective Worksheets. 10. Reflecting on Reflection. Index.

Jane Wood has been involved in reflective practice for the last 20 years. She keeps her own reflective journal and facilitates reflective practice workshops, seminars and monthly group sessions. She is a supervisor and teacher of reflective practice at the University of Westminster and is the head of practitioner development and reflective practice at the International School of Homeopathy, London. She lives in London, UK.

INSPIRING CREATIVE SUPERVISION
Caroline Schuck
and Jane Wood

Paperback: £17.99 / $28.95
ISBN: 978 1 84905 079 1
192 pages

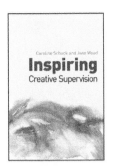

Creative supervision can be a stimulating and valuable alternative to questioning and discussion in the context of a supervision session. This book proposes using many different techniques and materials, as well as the rich experience of the imagination and the senses, and encourages the reader to go beyond the formal demands of their role, and feel inspired by creativity, spontaneity and experiential work.

The authors draw together theory, research and practical exercises, and provide ideas for setting up and running creative supervision sessions, including how to get started. The ideas and techniques outlined in this book include the use of narrative, drawings and visualisation, and the authors also clearly explain how to make the best use of props and resources such as toys, objet trouvé and picture postcards.

The innovative approach described in this book will be of interest to supervisors and non-supervisors alike. It will serve as a road map for expressive arts therapists, social workers, psychotherapists, psychologists and mental health and health care workers, and will also be an invaluable resource for other professionals such as teachers, mentors, coaches and human resources departments.

Contents: Introduction. 1. Introducing Creative Supervision. 2. Becoming a Creative Supervisor. 3. Opening up Unconscious Communication. 4. Using Toys and Bricks. 5. Discovering Visualization, Metaphor and Drawing. 6. Enjoying Limitless Resources. 7. Creating Narrative. 8. Using People as Props. 9. Developing an Inner Supervisor. 10. Beginnings, Endings, Ritual and Ceremony. 11. Working at a Distance. 12. Collecting and Making Resources and Props. References. Further Reading. Index.

Caroline Schuck is a qualified supervisor with a background in humanistic psychotherapy. She teaches supervision skills and reflective practice at the University of Westminster, works one to one, runs groups and co-facilitates supervision skills workshops for the London Deanery. **Jane Wood** has been involved in reflective practice for the last 20 years. She keeps her own reflective journal and facilitates reflective practice workshops, seminars and monthly group sessions. She is a supervisor and teacher of reflective practice at the University of Westminster and is the head of practitioner development and reflective practice at the International School of Homeopathy, London. She lives in London, UK.